# QUANTUM LONGEVITY

## By

### Paul Yanick, Jr., Ph.D. and Vincent C. Giampapa, M.D.

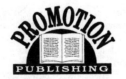

# QUANTUM LONGEVITY

### By
### *Paul Yanick, Jr., Ph.D. and Vincent C. Giampapa, M.D.*

#### Copyright © 1997 by Paul Yanick, Jr., Ph.D.

### PROMOTION PUBLISHING
### 3368 GOVERNOR DRIVE
### SUITE #144
### SAN DIEGO, CA 92122
### 1-800-231-1776

**Disclaimer:**
This book represents decades of scientific research and study in the fields of anatomy, physiology, biochemistry, pharmacology, endocrinology, neurology, nutrition, psychology, and functional medicine. In an effort to make this book less tedious, we have omitted thousands of scientific and textbook references from some of these specialized fields. The concepts presented in this book are indisputable facts of life that follow the laws of nature and are based on sound reasoning and common sense.

**Important Notice:**
If you have a disease or any type of health-related problem, you should consult with a medical physician. This book is not meant to replace a medical exam. The contents of this book are not meant to diagnose, prognosticate or render medical advice to people with medical conditions or diseases. It should be used in cooperation with your physician to solve your health problems. Its sole purpose is to increase nutritional awareness and to educate people regarding the laws of nature and life and to help individuals learn ways to improve their general health and well-being. In the event that you use this information on your own, you are prescribing for yourself, and the publisher and authors assume no responsibility.

#### ISBN# 1-57901-007-5
### PRINTED IN THE UNITED STATES OF AMERICA

# DEDICATIONS

This book is dedicated to my wife, Bonnie Lee whose insight, enthusiasm, love, and support made it possible for me to write it. It is further dedicated to my parents who provided me with love and taught me the values that resulted in my deep desire to help people conquer age-related illnesses.

**Paul Yanick**

I would like to dedicate this book to both my parents, Vincent and Lucy, for continually encouraging me to be an independent thinker; and to my wife, Susan, and children, Doug and Nina, for allowing me the time to walk my own path.

**Vincent C. Giampapa**

# ACKNOWLEDGMENTS

We thank Thomas Scott Yanick for his creative work with the graphic illustrations found in this book and Heather Rose Yanick for her help typing. We also want to thank the thousands of seminar participants who greatly encouraged us to undertake this project.

# TABLE OF CONTENTS

**Deliberately Left Blank**

# INTRODUCTION

A new kind of medicine is rapidly emerging: Anti-Aging Medicine. This medicine of the future has already taken a quantum leap toward understanding the deepest core of aging in the quantic or genetic realm of human functioning. Quantum Longevity explores the unimaginable frontiers of the microscopic secrets of genetic functioning. Achieving quantum longevity means activating anti-aging responses where aging begins—at the genetic level.

Millions of individuals who are striving for youth and longevity want anti-aging information and therapeutics. One in three adults under age 50 is now shopping for anti-aging hormones and nutritional products. Who doesn't want to live a longer, more productive life?

Anti-aging medicine is already helping individuals live longer, better lives than ever because of the many new hormone and nutritional therapies that keep arteries unclogged, blood pressure normal, aging bones from breaking, and eyesight and hearing from diminishing. Living to the age of 120 and beyond without the frailties of old age is no longer just a dream! Living our golden years with the health and vitality we had in our twenties and thirties is possible with anti-aging therapies.

Did you know that your physiological age can be younger—decades younger—than your chronological age?

Aging isn't just "getting older." It's a process that involves nutritional, emotional, and other biological changes that affect a person's overall health. A lack of exercise, relaxation and poor nutrition, are the wild cards that affect the speed of the aging process. Putting the brakes on the aging process means engaging in lifestyle changes that reverse aging in the quantic domain of human functioning.

Human aging is a result of the loss of proliferation capacity in normal cell populations of the body. Composed of some 100 trillion cells, anti-aging experts are now beginning to understand the mechanisms that control cell proliferation and renewal. In simple terms, these cells can be compared to a library with books that contain sentences and alphabetical letters. The chromosomes of cells are the books that fill the library, called the genome. DNA (short for deoxyribonucleic acid), found in the chromosomes, contains the written letters which are compiled in the sentence-like genes of our body. Containing instructions that would fill a thousand 600-page books, DNA acts like a contractor with a complete cabinet of blueprints for making all kinds of cells in the body.

Yet, there is much more to it. Each cell of your body constantly refers back to your biological library or genome, checking the blueprints printed there that allow you to proliferate, regenerate your body, and perform miraculous physiological functions. Minute by minute, this centralized genetic government, operating in the quantic domain of subatomic and molecular functioning, directs the body to repair damaged, broken down, and lost molecules in your cells. And as you will see, preserving these vital blueprints of human life is the key to extending the quantity and quality of your life to the point of achieving quantum longevity.

Humans are self-repairing: wounds heal, bones mend, and we recover from most illnesses.

At the molecular level our protein molecules are subject to continuous turnover. For example, youthful and healthy individuals replace the cells lining their intestines once every few days, those lining their urinary bladders once every two months, and red blood cells are replaced once every four months. This gene-based turnover of protein protects us from gene-damaging molecules that cause premature aging and allows the body to periodically replace all of it's cells. By speeding up normal cell proliferation and renewal functions while protecting the body's genetic master plan, we can avoid premature aging.

In the coming years, we know you will be hearing more about the human genome project. Sequencing an organism's genome—decoding, letter by letter, the message contained in it's genes—tells us exactly why and how aging occurs.

Scientists have exceeded all expectations and have already decoded over 30,000 of our estimated 80,000 genes. They have also estimated that 16 percent of these genes play a role in our metabolism, 12 percent are involved in cell to cell communication routines, and 4 percent help us and our cells reproduce.

Scientists are discovering new genes at a furious pace! Already, cataracts, obesity, prostate cancer, male infertility, schizophrenia, epilepsy, Alzheimer's disease, Usher Syndrome, breast cancer, and Rubinstein-Taybi Syndrome have been linked to genetic mutations. Since scientific knowledge is doubling every 3.5 years, we will have a 16 fold increase in our basic biological and technical knowledge by the year 2010. How can this knowledge benefit you?

The Longevity Institute International (LII) Anti-Aging Plan describes innovative methods that you can apply right now to preserve your genetic blueprints to the point of reaching your 100th birthday. Once you've accomplished this, you'll be first in line to benefit from new scientific discoveries of the future that may allow you to reach your 200th and even 300th birthday. As such, the LII Anti-Aging Plan bridges the gap between where science is today and where it will be in the future, giving you the opportunity to take advantage of all these anti-aging breakthroughs.

Our genetic blueprint is connected—directly or indirectly—to all functions and systems of our body. It is influenced in a positive or negative way by a kaleidoscopic array of factors: stress, diet, nutrition, exercise, and environmental toxins. Reaching the upper limits of our genetic potential is only possible when we integrate all these levels of quantum-genetic functioning into a comprehensive anti-aging plan—not from the intake of isolated synthetic hormones or drugs.

## BRIDGING THE GAP: THE LII ANTI-AGING PLAN

Along with a unique, revolutionary nutritional and anti-aging diet, LII uses nutraceutical-based hormone therapies that counteract the ravages of aging at all levels of genetic and hormonal functioning. But many anti-aging hormones are like a proverbial double-edged sword, since as many as 80 percent of these therapeutics are taken by the general public in excessive amounts. These single hormone-based approaches do not heal and fill the gaps in our genetic health and may cause serious disturbances in the quantic control of genetic mechanisms.

Aging is less a chronological marker than a combination of factors that determine the overall function of many systems of the body.

Most of us that develop an age-associated disorder do so because of a decline in the function of many organs and glands of the body. Some experts feel the immune system is also affected by aging, gradually losing its ability to defend us against outside threats—a virus, for example—and hence putting us at greater risk of illness.

Emotional and physiological issues have a major impact on the aging process. According to the American Psychiatric Association, 15 to 25 percent of elderly Americans suffer from age-related symptoms of dementia: memory loss, disorientation, and confusion. And, about another 20 percent of elderly Americans suffer from emotional disorders. All these types of disorders could have been prevented with early anti-aging medical intervention. It doesn't matter whether a person has mental illness, heart disease or arthritis, osteoporosis, or high blood pressure; anti-aging therapeutics can help rejuvenate organ systems—helping the body and mind function more efficiently.

An individual's chronological age need be no barrier! The LII Anti-Aging Plan provides health professionals and the interested general reader with basic anti-aging information as well as the latest findings in the field of anti-aging medicine. The fundamentals of anti-aging medicine are presented to give the reader a foundation, as well as a synopsis of verified research findings on ways to slow down—and in some cases—reverse the aging process.

The LII Anti-Aging Plan is unique and offers the most comprehensive physician designed, ongoing plan for anti-aging treatment. No other book combines anti-aging therapeutics with current research in a format for the health professional and general public. The authors have avoided oversimplification and the vagueness of popular anti-aging books on single hormone therapies—melatonin and DHEA, for example—while refraining from in-depth biochemical explanations for anti-aging therapies.

Interest in longevity has proliferated since the dawn of man. Anti-aging medicine as a science, however, is new and novelty breeds faddism. Health professionals need to separate fact from fiction to determine the best anti-aging treatment for their patients. Every magazine designed for the general reader includes articles on DHEA, melatonin, Human Growth Hormone (HGH), and the latest claims for anti-aging herbs and nutritional factors. This deluge of printed material is full of conflicting reports, beliefs, and opinions regarding guidelines for optimal health and longevity. The role of anti-aging medicine in increasing human lifespan has been extensively researched by LII scientists.

For the past decade, the LII has collected an enormous amount of medical data for the key facts of greatest concern to the individual in search of longevity. Now, to meet the needs of these individuals, we have arranged these facts in a format designed to provide you guidelines for maximum health and quantum longevity.

Although anti-aging medical experts can often work miracles with advanced technology and sophisticated nutrient delivery systems, they still need the help of the patient to make most treatments work. No matter how effective the anti-aging therapy, it will likely prove worthless if the patient's lifestyle promotes accelerated aging.

We have written this book to share with you the cutting-edge ideas and practices of the LII Anti-Aging Plan. Together we will explore and learn about the amazing capacity each of our bodies possesses to reverse the aging process. More importantly, you will learn how to expand and improve the quality of your life; not merely through the absence of disease but through the vitality and aliveness that you experienced when you were young.

This book is designed as a guidebook, an ongoing course in anti-aging therapeutics. It is designed to help you discover your unique and untapped potential for rejuvenation and a longer, healthier life. It provides you with the essential state-of-the-art information that LII teaches to patients and doctors in many international seminars and workshops.

Men and women following this informative report began to feel significantly better within weeks. Within a month they looked better, felt supercharged with energy, and slept more soundly at night. After 6-8 months, their skin wrinkled less, they got fewer colds, fewer aches and pains, and they lost weight.

The LII Anti-Aging Plan takes you behind the scenes as world-respected scientists...

◆ PREDICT future discoveries of stunning new cures for all age-related disorders.

◆ CONFRONT aging as a treatable disorder.

◆ PROBE our awe-inspiring and miraculous body for explanations to why and how we age.

◆ EXAMINE the scientific forces and factors that cause the body to age prematurely.

◆ PRESENT proven clinical methods that you can apply now to brake accelerated aging processes.

Based on solid scientific research, LII's Anti-Aging Plan uses the most up-to-date information available to provide safe, medically approved, balanced anti-aging hormonal and nutritional guidelines to give you added years of healthy life. For the first time, the LII Anti-Aging Plan offers you a comprehensive plan to preserve and restore your genetic blueprint, a plan that can enhance the quality and length of your life—and even save your life.

Now LII has placed all of these authoritative facts at your personal disposal through the LII Anti-Aging Plan.

Should I take this hormone or vitamin? Is there any reason it might be dangerous for me? What about possible side effects and interactions with other hormones and nutritional factors? What are the best anti-aging hormone and nutritional therapies available to me? The answers to all these questions can now be at your fingertips—presented in concise, easy-to-understand language. For the long and healthy life that each member of your family deserves, the LII Anti-Aging Plan offers the most advanced and comprehensive guide to current anti-aging therapies.

**PAUL YANICK, JR., PH.D.**

*Medical Research Director, Longevity Institute International*

**VINCENT C. GIAMPAPA, M.D.**

*Founder and President, Longevity Institute International*

*Vice President, American Academy of Anti-Aging Medicine*

# CHAPTER 1

# QUANTUM LONGEVITY AND THE LII ANTI-AGING PLAN

Imagine if someone had told you twenty—or even ten-years ago that there was a way you could slow down the aging process. With good reason, it would have sounded farfetched. Because until the last ten years or so, aging was considered inevitable.

At long last, medical science has proven that aging is a treatable condition. Recent advances in medical research have led to a growing perception that what is perceived as the "natural" mental and physical decline associated with human aging is delayable, preventable, and in some cases, reversible.[1-11]

The coalescing of modern therapies and preventive regimens into a comprehensive science of anti-aging medicine is only now beginning to occur. Today it is widely agreed that most individuals can benefit greatly from an in depth analysis of their metabolic status followed by the administration of a comprehensive program of targeted vitamin, nutrient, hormone and drug therapies.

## AGING CAN BE MANAGED

At LII, we recognize that aging is not a simple chronological event, but a complex interaction of specific dysfunctions of the body. Symptoms of aging can be identified at the organic, cellular, molecular and chromosomal levels. Ideally, each may be targeted by an appropriate, individualized treatment strategy. However, the LII Anti-Aging Plan provides you with a multi-faceted attack on the very mechanisms of human aging. These therapies are designed to slow down the aging process by balancing our cell's chemical and molecular environment or our "cellular soup."

## LIFE SPAN AND LIFE EXPECTANCY

Life span refers to how long a human being can live when utilizing the body's maximum genetic potential. The potential human life span is at least 120 years old. How do we know this? Scientists have documented that some humans are presently living to the age of 120 and beyond. Life expectancy refers to the average length of life a person actually lives within their respective culture or country. In the United States and most industrialized countries, this averages approximately 76 years. Why such a discrepancy between the potential of 120 years and the average life expectancy of 76 years?

The vast majority of us do not reach our full life span potential because of environmental toxins, infectious diseases, and disorders of premature aging involving damage to our genes. Genetic damage involves changes in the normal sequence of chemicals called nucleotides with our genes. The LII Anti-Aging Plan targets the cell's elegant genetic world—protecting genes from damage.

## REVITALIZING YOUR CELLULAR SOUP

Let's start with a basic understanding of "cellular soup." In and around our cells are molecules, nutrients and chemicals that determine our genetic potential. The amount of nutrients in this cellular soup depends on a variety of factors: illness (which depletes vital nutrients), diet (maldigestion or poor diets provide suboptimal levels of nutrients), drug use (tobacco, recreational drugs, prescription medications, and alcohol destroy these nutrients), and stress (which depletes nutrients required by the body to make anti-aging hormones).

With advancing age, our cellular soup accumulates damage and cellular waste material caused by destructive molecular predators called free radicals. These molecular predators destroy cell walls and DNA, causing all the consequences of premature molecular and tissue aging.

The good news is that supplementation with anti-aging nutrients can counteract the negative effects of illness, diet, drug use, stress, and destroy free radicals. These powerful nutrients in your body's cellular soup are what allow you to think, feel, perform, and look youthful and healthy.

People with seemingly boundless energy enjoy the vitality and stamina that can come only when their cellular soup is rich in nutrients and free from molecular predators.

## EFFECTIVE ANTI-AGING WEIGHT LOSS!

LII has developed a weight loss plan that makes it easy for you to reach and stay at your ideal weight. By improving the balance of pH, hormones, and biochemicals, this plan forces your body to lose body fat. Even if you fasted or tried other diet plans and failed, this diet plan works to shed unwanted body fat. Unlike the ZONE diet that only addresses the insulin/glucagon balance or calorie-counting diets, the LII Anti-Aging Diet works by recharging your cellular soup and correcting the genetic, chemical, and hormonal causes of being overweight.

You'll be able to eat three full meals a day without experiencing gnawing hunger pains or food cravings. Unlike many fad diets, LII also promotes optimal weight loss by boosting your body's natural production of HGH and IGF-1—hormones that burn fat and build muscles. Based on over two decades of clinical research, this diet plan allows you to lose weight effectively and permanently.

## STOPPING YOUR AGING CLOCKS

The decline in the ebb and flow of hormones and genetic potential with advancing age provides dramatic evidence of aging clocks in action. When these aging clocks tick too fast, they accelerate the pathways of aging, causing the body to lose its ability to repair damage from environmental factors. This process produces chaotic changes in our cells, tissues, and organs. **Figure 1** depicts the three aging clocks addressed by the LII Anti-Aging Plan:

1   The pineal gland which acts as our <u>central aging clock</u>. Its messenger, melatonin travels to the peripheral clock inside the cell. It knows how old we are—and signals many glands to shut down as we age.

2   The <u>peripheral clock</u>, located in the cell's nucleus, activates energy-producing mitochondria of the cells to provide fuel for genetic functions.

3   The <u>telomere clock</u>, located on the DNA-containing chromosomes, which controls the life span of our cells.

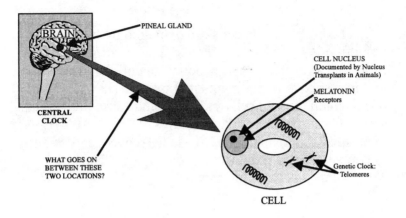

**Figure 1.** The Aging Clocks.

## AGING THEORIES

It is a misconception that the damaging effects of aging are inevitable. Remarkable breakthroughs in modern science and medicine have proven that aging can be properly managed. The truth is, our biological age can be decades less than our actual chronological age.

The foundation for LII's successful administration of the Anti-Aging Plan lies with the understanding of the key aging theories. They are the Free Radical Theory, Wear and Tear Theory, Neuroendocrine Theory, and Genetic Control Theory. Most scientists agree that all of these theories offer some insight into the aging process. The LII Anti-Aging Plan addresses all these theories of aging.

## FREE RADICAL THEORY

The body and its cells are damaged by biochemical compounds called free radicals. These compounds are produced as normal waste products of cellular metabolism and in response to environmental toxins. They are highly reactive and toxic to cells and DNA and cause our cellular soup to become depleted in nutrients. The LII Anti-Aging Plan utilizes antioxidants and free radial scavengers designed to counteract and minimize the damaging effects of these compounds on our cellular soup.

## WEAR AND TEAR THEORY

The body and its cells are damaged by overuse and abuse. This destruction occurs at both the cellular and organ levels. The LII Anti-Aging Plan seeks to stimulate the body's own maintenance and replacement process by augmenting immune system and repair function mechanisms deep within the molecular biology of our cellular soup.

## NEUROENDOCRINE THEORY

The body's maintenance function (repair and regulating systems) are damaged as key hormones drop to low levels. Two of these key hormones: Human Growth Hormone (HGH) and Insulin-like Growth Factor (IGF-1) cause the aging process to accelerate as they decline. The LII Anti-Aging Plan uses advanced nutrient delivery systems along with hormone precursor nutrients to re-establish the synchronicity of the entire neuroendocrine system and elevate HGH and IGF-1 hormone levels to help reset the hormonal regulatory systems necessary for optimal health and vitality.

## GENETIC CONTROL THEORY

The body and its cells are genetically programmed to stop repair and maintenance after a fixed period of time. This control is coded into the DNA blueprints of body's cells. The LII Anti-Aging Plan slows the biological clock by augmenting the basic building blocks of DNA in the cell. Therefore, less damage to DNA may occur on a daily basis and DNA repair may be enhanced.

The LII Anti-Aging Plan incorporates vitamins, minerals, nutraceuticals (plant-derived hormone precursors), hormones, anti-aging foods and a breakthrough protein product that boosts the production of HGH and IGF-1 in the body and other lifestyle factors to:

1) Protect the body's cellular soup and DNA from harmful free radicals.

2) Eliminate the "wear and tear" of stress.

3) Enhance the body's natural production and activity of hormones.

4) Enhance and balance neurotransmitters and brain function.

5) Keep the immune, digestive, and other systems of the body functioning at youthful levels.

6) Augment the body's ability to repair DNA damage while enhancing the rate of cell repair and maintenance so that the cell renews itself at the genetic level and produces the nucleotides and polypeptides to maximize cellular function and renewal.

Today's dramatic advances in anti-aging diagnostics and therapies allow for a sophisticated and multileveled assessment of individual's biological age. The relative

7

risk of future health problems may be determined, as well as identification of genetic age and some genetically determined disease processes at the cellular level. Biomedical interventions, including appropriate pharmacological and therapeutic measures and nutritional regimes can thus be implemented and monitored to forestall the onset of age-related mental and physical deterioration. LII's basic program is three-fold:

1. **Measure Aging Levels** - Utilizing LII's unique Biomarker Matrix Protocol™, the aging rate is measured on four levels: overall body function, skin analysis, molecular analysis and DNA analysis.

2. **Treatment** - A number of treatment regimens are available to counteract the effects of aging. Based on individual data processed by the Biomarker Testing Computer Profile, these regimens simultaneously act to inhibit the aging process at every observable level.

3. **Monitor** - Because the treatment is both complex and dynamic, periodic re-evaluation and adjustment of the prescribed regimen is an integral part of the LII program. Most individuals are re-tested at six to twelve month intervals for assessment of treatment results and adjustment of the anti-aging regimen as needed.


Today, LII is at the forefront of the exciting field of anti-aging medicine, offering the most comprehensive plan for anti-aging. LII's growing network of physician's utilizes the emerging technologies of genetic engineering, biotechnology and molecular biology to combat the aging process not only on the physical level, but also down to the very deepest quantic domain of life: the chromosome and DNA itself.

Protecting and effecting this "blueprint" level of life is a cornerstone of the LII program. Augmenting the body's ability to repair DNA damage by improving the nutrient and molecular content of our cellular soup; as well as stimulating the immune system and keeping the neurohormonal centers of the body functioning more efficiently are key components in retarding the aging process.

Already, LII has documented measurable improvements in:

1) mental speed and clarity

2) skin tightness and moisture

3) libido and sexual function

4) general mood and energy levels

5) immune functions

6) muscle strength and endurance

7) bone density and strength

8) exercise and aerobic capacity


The attentive reader of this book will recognize that the LII Anti-Aging Plan forms an intelligent alternative to accepting illness as part and parcel of the aging process. If anyone reading this book finds portions of it too difficult to understand, they will do better by skipping over the technical explanations and carefully reviewing the "POINTS TO REMEMBER" and "WHAT YOU CAN DO NOW" sections at the end of each chapter.

The answer to the fundamental question "does the LII Anti-Aging Plan work?" is "yes", and we believe that this modern, safe strategy for reversing human aging will provide you with a broad spectrum of exciting, health-enhancing possibilities. LII's approach extends the period of what we now call "middle age" from the 35-55 range to the 35-70 age group.

When our bodies maintain their youthful physiology we will be virtually free of many of the diseases that now plague mankind! Quantum Longevity is the first book that describes innovative and effective ways to preserve your body's biomolecular integrity at the genetic level of cellular functioning: your genetic blueprint. Every person—young, middle-aged, or old—will benefit from this comprehensive approach to extending the human life span.

## ACTIVATING QUANTUM HEALING AND REGENERATION

Beyond the visible world of atoms, molecules, and chemicals are subatomic particles which physicists call biophotons. Biophotons are impulses of energy that arrange molecular structures and play a vital role in getting nutrients into our cellular soup. These invisible energies silently orchestrate, instruct, guide, and govern genetic processes with unfaltering exactitude, giving our body a myriad of functions.

Scientists have already shown that our thoughts and attitudes can be transformed into molecules. Every thought or attitude you have sends a biophoton message to the cellular world—altering chemicals and hormone activity.

Without going into great detail, energetic mechanisms are the underlying control systems that regulate anti-aging mechanisms. As anti-aging physicians move toward this new pathway and understanding of the aging process, we come closer to grasping the reality that integrates life and energy in the human organism.

Our Level 5 biomarker test assesses the quantum domain of human aging. And, to correct aging in this dimension, we will introduce you to a new concept of nutrition: Quantum Nutrition. Individuals taking Quantum Nutrition report that they feel more energetic, healthier and sexier than they have since their youth. Quantum Nutrition actually corrects and reverses much of the "wear and tear" that occurs in our bodies as we age.

In the next chapter, you'll assess your own unique biomarker status. Then, you can apply our Quantum Nutritional regimen and anti-aging diet to:

A. **Preserve our Genetic Blueprint by Limiting Damage to DNA** - Antioxidants and free radical scavengers are used to limit the damaged DNA replication process and reduce compounds which can disrupt and destroy cellular/mitochondrial DNA.

B. **Enhance DNA Synthesis** - Nutrients are used to increase the rate of cell repair and maintenance, allowing the cell to renew itself on a genetic level. This renewal at the genetic level produces nucleotides and polypeptides needed to maximize cellular function and regeneration.

C. **Stimulate and augment the immune system** - Enhancing natural immunological mechanisms enables the body to continually fight off attacks by microbes and environmental toxins.

## BRIDGING THE GAP: WHAT THE FUTURE HOLDS

The next few decades will provide us with medical miracles that promise to extend human life span to the age of 130. In about 30-40 years, living to the age of 150 and beyond will be a definite reality. By preserving your genetic blueprint and nourishing your cellular soup with Quantum Nutrition, the LII Anti-Aging Plan outlined in this book may extend your life span by 30 years or more. This would translate into your living your last three decades with a high-level health and well-being...and, by that time anti-aging scientists will have discovered methods to extend your life another 20 or 30 years.

Preserving and restoring your genetic blueprint so that the least amount of damage occurs in the next decade, will allow you to take advantage of the quantum changes that will be available in the field of anti-aging medicine. The LII Anti-Aging Plan bridges the gap between where science is today and where it will be inevitably in the next few decades, giving you the opportunity to take full advantage of all the miraculous advances available at that time.

The LII Anti-Aging Plan provides you with easy, safe, inexpensive solutions that could well be the healing miracles you have been searching for. Healing miracles that lead to quantum longevity. You will be stunned when you see for yourself just how powerful this breakthrough anti-aging plan is. Tap into the world's most effective anti-aging protocol for reversal of aging, taming stress, increasing energy, restoring memory, reducing body fat, invigorating a stagnant libido, and looking your absolute best: The LII Anti-Aging Plan.

If you are willing to make the simple lifestyle changes and commit yourself to living a longer and healthier life, you truly can stop the aging clocks. There is no need to live your older years with diminished vigor and degenerative diseases. Set a goal now to live your retirement with youthful energy—the way you did when you were younger!

Life is so precious! Good health and vitality can be realized whether you are 30 or 80. Now is the time to take the first steps in revitalizing your body through the LII Anti-Aging Plan. Get on the road to an enhanced quality of life!

KEY POINTS TO REMEMBER...

◆ Aging is not a simple chronological event, but a complex interaction of many different dysfunctions of the body.

◆ The LII Biomarker Matrix Protocol™ can identify symptoms of aging at the organic, cellular, molecular, and chromosomal levels.

◆ The LII Anti-Aging Plan provides you with a multi-faceted attack on all the mechanisms of aging.

◆ A youthful metabolism has a lot to do with HGH and IGF-1 levels. These extraordinary hormones with their vast and truly astonishing scope of health benefits control the ebb and flow of the anti-aging mechanisms in the body and have the power to regenerate and extend life.

WHAT YOU CAN DO NOW

◆ Determine your need for this plan by taking the LII Biomarker Self-Test in the following chapter of this book. Make a copy of this test and use it as a means of monitoring your progress on the LII Anti-Aging Plan.

♦   Set a goal to lower your biological age by 10, 20, or 30 years below your chronological age.

♦   As you read through this book, take notes on points that have a particular application to your own personal lifestyle and prepare a grocery list of foods that will lower your risks for heart disease, stroke, and other age-related diseases.

# CHAPTER 2

## DETERMINING YOUR BIOMARKER LEVELS

Today's medical science allows us to determine our body's biological age. The technology which determines the degree of age-related impairment at the physiological, cellular, molecular, and genetic levels is called "Biomarker Analysis."

Biomarker Analysis is in essence, an in-depth physical and health examination. Each person provides their doctor with a detailed physical health, lifestyle, and genetic history. Further tests are proscribed and may be done on samples of an individual's blood, urine, tissue, and hair. The data gathered through this systemic look at a person's "age" is processed, analyzed, and treatment regimens are recommended that can help to inhibit the aging process.

One of the key advantages of LII's program is its unique individual measuring system which profiles the body's aging clock and indicates where aging damage is occurring. LII uses its designed and patented "biomarker" tests to identify potential problem areas and treat them before damage occurs. Biomarkers are enzymes, skin cells, and biochemicals produced by the body. The biomarker tests provide the earliest indication of when a body is approaching the critical aging juncture.

Biomarkers are also predictive of the individual's risk of developing age-related diseases or illnesses. A synthesis of modern science and digital information processing has provided the possibility of performing a comprehensive, computer-aided biomarker screening to determine an individual's biological age (i.e. the overall body as well as its individual organ systems), and to predict the impending obstacles to maintaining a healthy and productive mental and physical state.

## DETERMINING YOUR BIOMARKERS

Age can be deceiving. There are some people who look and feel much younger than their chronological age. And, there are some people who look and feel much older. No matter what a person's age, there is something they can do to prevent the mental decline and physical damage caused by aging.

**Figure 2** illustrates what happens when we age prematurely. The decline in pituitary-secreted HGH, which declines steadily as we age, robs us of our youth. Our research shows that when HGH is increased through the LII Anti-Aging Plan, it affects every cell in the body, bringing many physiological functions back to youthful levels. HGH is converted to another anti-aging hormone in the liver called IGF-1. When plasma IGF-1 levels increase, individuals report an extraordinary range of age-reversing effects: energy levels increase, sexual performance is enhanced, blood circulation and pressure normalizes, immunity is enhanced, hair regrows, wrinkles are removed or decreased, skin becomes thicker and softer, cellulite is eliminated, memory improves, vision and hearing improve, fat decreases, muscle mass increases, digestion improves, and bones are strengthened.

The LII Anti-Aging Plan focuses on the most powerful dimensions of natural healing: boosting HGH and IGF-1, strengthening the body's immune system; stress reduction; diet improvement; and lifestyle change. Symptoms of accelerated aging are varied and numerous, ranging from a lack of energy to joint stiffness or muscle pain. The only way you know for certain if you are aging

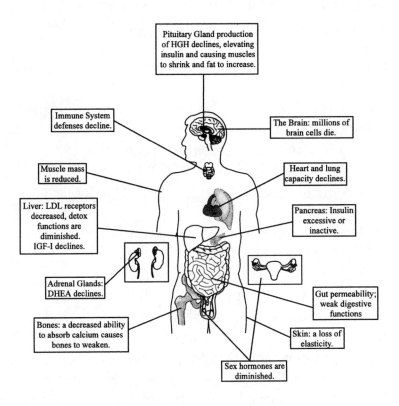

**Figure 2.** What happens when we age.

17

too fast is too have the Biomarker Matrix Protocol™ by LII-trained physicians. However, the following questionnaire will give you a general sense of your need to alter your biological age with the LII Anti-Aging Plan:

1. Do you have reduced lean body mass?
2. Do you have increased body fat?
3. Do you lack a positive sense of well being?
4. Do you have reduced energy and vitality?
5. Is your waist measurement greater than it was ten years ago?
6. Is your hip measurement greater than it was ten years ago?
7. Do you notice reduced muscle strength over the past ten years?
8. Do you notice a reduced ability to exercise?
9. Do you notice increased levels of depression?
10. Do you feel increased levels of anxiety over the past decade?
11. Do you have reduced mental performance over the past decade?
12. Do you feel stressed-out at times?
13. Are you generally pessimistic about life?
14. Are you quick to get angry?
15. Do you have difficulty focusing and concentrating?
16. Do you look older than people your age?
17. Do you feel tired when you wake up in the morning?
18. Are you less social than in the past?
19. Have you noticed a decline in your sexual performance?
20. Do you have trouble sleeping?

21. Does it take longer for you to fall asleep?
22. Do you have more difficulty thinking clearly and remembering?
23. Do you have a decreased HDL cholesterol?
24. Do you have an increased LDL cholesterol?
25. Do you have a deficiency in DHEA or melatonin?
26. Has your vision diminished over the past decade?
27. Has your hearing diminished over the past decade?
28. Does it take a long time for you to get over a cold or flu?
29. Does it take a long time for cuts or bruises to heal?
30. Is your blood pressure borderline or high?
31. Do you suffer from indigestion?
32. Do you often fail to have regular bowel movements?
33. Do you get up at night to urinate?
34. Are you slowly losing your hair?
35. Do you have food or inhalant allergies?
36. Do you have white spots on your fingernails?
37. Do you have longitudinal ridges on your fingernails?
38. Do your fingernails appear thin and weak?
39. Do you have more headaches than a decade ago?
40. Do you have cold hands or feet?

If you answered "yes" to more than ten of these questions, your biological age is the same or greater than your chronological age. If you've answered "yes" to more that half these questions, there is a large gap between your biological age and your chronological age—indicating your body is aging too fast. Ideally, we want to set a goal to lower our biological age by 10, 20, and even 30 years below our chronological age.

## How To Measure Your Own Biomarkers At Home

For your convenience, we designed the LII Biomarker Self-Test: a test you can take in the privacy of your own home. Although not as comprehensive as the LII Biomarker Matrix Protocol, this unique test allows you to assess your own unique biomarker levels. With these tests results, you will be in a position to monitor your own progress on the LII Anti-Aging Plan. In brief, these tests assess your body composition, reaction time, visual acuity, flexibility, body fat percentages, and lean muscle mass.

For readers seeking more specific biomarker testing, anti-aging physicians are listed in the Appendix B of this book. In addition to the LII Anti-Aging Plan, these LII-trained physicians will use the Biomarker Matrix Protocol™, designed by LII, to determine your rate of aging and to prescribe targeted therapies and personalized treatment programs.

You'll learn more about this revolutionary tool for anti-aging medicine and other LII cutting-edge technological advances that help protect the body from the effects of aging in Chapter 11.

LII physicians use biomarkers to reset your genetic code and slow down or stop your aging clocks. The result: your body functions at more youthful levels.

# THE LII BIOMARKER SELF-TEST

Name ————————————————————————

Age———————— Date ————————————————

## TEST 1: PHYSICAL FACTORS

### (INSTRUCTIONS FOUND IN APPENDIX B):

Percent Body Fat: ————————  ————————  ————————

*Ideal -0 points--Borderline-4 points-- Abnormal - 8 points*

Weight: ————————  ————————  ————————  ————————

*Ideal +10lbs 4 points   +20lbs 6 points   >30lbs 10 points*

Skin Elasticity Test:         ————————————    ————————————

*Normal-0 points          Abnormal-4 points*

Static Balance Test:          ————————————    ————————————

*Normal-0 points          Abnormal-4 points*

## TEST 2: RATE EACH OF THE FOLLOWING PHYSICAL SYMPTOMS ACCORDINGLY:

**Scale**: 0 = Never, 1 = Occasionally have mild symptoms, 2 = Occasionally have moderate to severe symptoms, 3 = Frequently have mild symptoms, 4 = Frequently have moderate to severe symptoms.

## A. Gut Biomarkers :

___ Nausea or vomiting ___ Diarrhea ___ Constipation ___ Bloated feeling ___ Belching or passing gas ___ Heartburn ___ Bad breath ____ Intolerance to fatty foods ____ Light or clay-colored stools ____ Dark Urine ____ Bitter taste in mouth ____ Food allergies

## B. Metabolic Biomarkers:

___ Fatigue, sluggishness ___ Apathy, lethargy ___ Hyperactivity ___ Restlessness ____ Reduced vitality ____ Increased body fat

21

___ Overweight ___ Abnormal Waist/Hip ratio ___ Abnormal Muscle/Fat Ratio ____ Abnormal skin elasticity tests

## C. Hormonal Biomarkers:

____Excessive fatigue ___Weakness ___ Nervousness/irritability ___ Mental depression ___ Inability to concentrate ___ Moments of confusion ___ Poor memory ___ Feelings of frustration ___ Light-headedness ___Dizziness that occurs upon standing___Low blood pressure___Insomnia___Premenstrual tension___Craving for sweets___Headaches___Alcohol intolerance___Low Blood Sugar ___ Excessive hunger ___ Palpitation ___ Poor resistance to infections ___Food and/or inhalant allergies ___ Low body temperature ___ Unexplained hair loss ___ Difficulty building muscle___Difficulty gaining weight___Tendency to inflammation

## D. Skin Biomarkers:

_____ Dry and thin skin ____ Itchy skin ____ Scanty perspiration ____ Acne ___ Hives, rashes ____ Hair Loss ____ Excessive sweating

## E. Mental Biomarkers:

___ Poor Memory ___ Confusion, poor comprehension ___ Poor concentration ____ Poor physical coordination ___ Learning difficulties ____ Depressed ____ Anxiety

## F. Muscle/Joint Biomarkers:

____ Pain or aches in joints ___ Arthritis ___ Muscle aches or pains ___ Joint stiffness ___ Reduced muscle strength ____ Reduced exercise performance ____ Reduced lean body mass

## G. Head Biomarkers:

____Watery or itchy eyes___Itchy ears___Ringing in ears/hearing loss ___ Bags or dark circles under eyes ___ Swollen, reddened eyes ___ Vision loss ___Dizziness ___ Sinus problems ___ Stuffy nose ____ Inhalant Allergies ____ Tongue coated white or brown ___ Dental problems ___ Gum irritations

Total Test 1 Score =_____ Total Test 2 Score = _____
Grand Total = _____

*Scores in the range 30-60 may indicate early signs of premature aging.*
*Scores in the range 61-100 may indicate moderate signs of premature aging.*
*Scores greater than 100 may indicate advanced states of premature aging.*

## STARTING THE LII ANTI-AGING PLAN

The body experiences changes as we grow older. But time alone is not responsible for eroding health. This means the damaging effect of age may not be inevitable. The LII Anti-Aging Plan strives to prevent age-associated ailments and diseases. Prevention is important because many individuals adapt to less-than-optimal health without realizing it. By starting the LII Anti-Aging Plan you will lower your risks of heart disease, stroke, and other age-related disorders.

Without a doubt, the LII Anti-Aging Plan will bring you closer to understanding the causes of accelerated aging. Scientists have discovered certain genetic and biochemical factors that are linked to accelerated aging and anti-aging mechanisms of the body. Certain lifestyles, diets, and habits contribute to the development of age-related disorders. LII has enough research on hand to support the exciting prospect that you have some degree of control over the aging process. By eliminating or reducing certain factors that place you at risk for age-related illnesses, and by then striving to include anti-aging hormones, nutrients, and foods in your diets, you greatly increase our chances of preventing—or possibly surviving—age-related diseases.

The next four chapters will explain how LII's successful administration of the Anti-Aging Plan lies with the understanding of the key aging theories (Wear and Tear Theory, Free Radical Theory, Neuroendocrine Theory, and Genetic Control Theory). By applying the knowledge gained in these chapters and following the Anti-Aging Diet and Quantum Nutritional Plan (Chapters 8 and 9), you can add decades to your years. However, this knowledge is worthless if you don't apply it in your daily life routines.

## POINTS TO REMEMBER....

♦ Your Biomarker status will change on the LII Anti-Aging Plan about once every six to eight weeks. Make copies of the test form and continue taking the LII Biomarker Self-Test until your scores indicate you have halted or reversed premature aging in your body.

♦ The age-defying effects of HGH can resculpt the body by reducing fat and increasing muscle strength, and smooth out facial wrinkles, restore skin elasticity and thickness, revive sexuality, elevate moods and lift the spirits, giving you superior mental and physical performance.

♦ Boosting HGH and IGF-1 while preserving your genetic blueprint are the primary goals of the LII Anti-Aging Plan.

## WHAT YOU CAN DO NOW

♦ Take the LII Biomarker Self-Test.

♦ Repeat this test every 6-8 weeks to monitor your progress on the LII Anti-Aging Plan.

♦ Set realistic goals to change your lifestyle and follow the LII Anti-Aging Plan.

♦ Customize these goals to fit your needs and current lifestyle.

♦ Replace smoking or overeating with a daily exercise program.

♦ Changes are easy to make on a long-term basis. When you make small but permanent changes in your lifestyle.

# CHAPTER 3

## PREVENTING STRESS-INDUCED WEAR AND TEAR

According to the wear and tear theory of aging, the body and its cells are damaged by overuse and abuse. This destruction occurs at the quantum-genetic, cellular and organ levels. Stress causes a "wearing out" of the vital organs and glands of the body. This wear and tear erodes and disrupts the normal genetic, molecular, and biochemical routines of cells, tissues, organs, and speeds up our aging clocks.

A large proportion of health care costs are devoted to treating stress-related diseases which are caused by faulty lifestyle habits. In fact, 75 percent of the premature deaths in this country are due to lifestyle-related degenerative diseases such as cardiovascular disease and cancer.[1] So, the astounding truth is prevention is essentially in our hands.

### ARE YOU EXPERIENCING STRESS SYMPTOMS?

Anxiety and stress have long been known to bring on many symptoms and diseases. In fact, some people feel that the sharp rise in age-related disorders may be due to a more intense—and stressful—work related environment. Constant stress—or a panicked way of dealing with stress—may aggravate a multitude of symptoms.

Recognizing the most common symptoms of stress is the first step in taking the edge off stress. It's important to be aware that these symptoms serve as early warning signals to alert us that our lifestyle needs to be altered. Evaluate your stress symptoms. See how many of the following common stress symptoms you have:

| | |
|---|---|
| Caffeine/sugar addictions | Insomnia |
| Fatigue | Impatience |
| Anxiety | Cold sweats |
| Forgetfulness | Dry mouth |
| Headaches or lightheadedness | Overeating |
| Inability to concentrate | Irritability |
| Constipation or Diarrhea | Waking up tired |
| Shallow/rapid breathing | Apathy |
| Tightness in chest | Anger |
| Jaw clenching or teeth grinding | Rapid pulse |
| Depression | Pounding heart |
| End of the day exhaustion | |

If you are experiencing 6 or more of these symptoms, now is the time to initiate a method of stress control—relaxation techniques, deep breathing, aerobic exercise, biofeedback—that will help reduce the negative effects of stress.

If your boss is continually on your case or traffic jams make you angry or make your stomach tight, you had better learn how to manage your anger. Rather than blow your stack and increase dangerous stress symptoms, why not take the following steps:

Breathe and Wait. Before you say or do anything, take a series of deep breaths giving your anger a chance to pass or at least cool down.

Analyze the situation. If your anger is ready to boil over, try to tune out by focusing on something relaxing or pleasurable. Make yourself aware of how anger is a dangerous emotion that can be very harmful to your body. Try to realize how this destructive emotion accomplishes nothing and often makes you look foolish and say things you don't really mean.

## THE WEAR AND TEAR OF STRESS

Alarmingly, Americans make 187 million visits to the doctor a year for stress-related symptoms. In this modern day life, stress has become a major part of life. Unfortunately, when stress becomes part of the daily routine, the body begins to age at an accelerated rate.

The aging of the body is an active process. Lifestyle determines how the aging process takes its toll in the accumulated loss of the genetic blueprint as well as mental and physical functions.

Increased vulnerability to illness as we age is a direct result of how we live our lives. At this point, you might ask, "How do I prevent stress-related aging?"

A big percentage of what we do in our lives is going to cause unwanted stress. Rather than ignoring the problem and allowing leisure time to get pushed aside, we need to find the time to exercise, relax, and eat foods that provide our bodies with what it needs to unwind and tone down the damaging effects of stress in our lives.

In most cases, the biggest stress factor is our diet. Diet-induced stress causes blood sugar levels and hormones to go up and down like a roller coaster. And even though we may not initially feel the effects of diet-induced stress, research has demonstrated it can take a major toll on the body.

The hormones released by stress eat at the digestive tract and weaken the heart, leading to both stroke and heart disease. The biochemical attacks brought about by the wrong dietary choices ultimately break down one's entire immune system and disrupt the delicate balance of our cellular soup, increasing the risks for deadly diseases.

How each individual copes with stress determines the rate of wear and tear or aging in the body. The fact of the matter is, we all experience stress and need to implement precautionary measures today, before it takes a serious toll on our bodies.

Simple changes in diet and lifestyle may well be our best weapons against stress-related diseases. The LII Anti-Aging Diet Plan has been found exceptionally effective in minimizing and controlling unpredictable bursts of emotional energy caused by tension, anxiety, anger and the generalized patterns of stress. The LII Quantum Nutritional Plan contains a combination of nutrients which are the dietary precursors to anti-stress and anti-aging hormones and neurotransmitter production in the body. These nutritional factors help to relax the body while providing it with special forms of easy-to-digest protein.

Why is protein so important?

When stress increases, the body's protein needs also increase. Excessive sugars in our diet damage or "cross-link" proteins that the pituitary gland uses to produce HGH and IGF-1 making them useless. The accumulation of these damaged, cross-linked proteins obstructs the passage of nutrients and waste between cells and subsequently damages our genes. In addition, the hormones insulin and glucagon are maintained in perfect balance with protein and adequate amounts of HGH and IGF-1 in our circulatory system.

But, here's the primary problem: Stress also breaks down body protein at an amazing rate. When the diet is low in easy-to-assimilate forms of bio-available protein, the body resorts to cannibalistic utilization of protein from both the gut and liver. This "wear and tear" stress reaction leeches the body's supply of protein causing ulcers, gallstones, functional liver disorders, leaky gut syndromes, and numerous other age-related disorders.

Prolonged stress also damages our gene-repairing mechanisms. Stress tears down molecules and parts of our cells. However, the process of repair and molecular rebuilding is written in our genes. Your cells always cross check your genetic blueprint for instructions that allow the body to rapidly repair stress-induced damage.

How is the information in your genetic blueprint transmitted to stress-worn parts of your body?

Like copying information from your computer onto a disk, the information is copied from DNA to RNA. The RNA-stored information is then delivered to tiny cellular factories called ribosomes. These ribosomes are then instructed to build three different kinds of proteins:

1   Structural proteins that are like the framework of a house

2   Signaling proteins that act like the telephone in your home needed to call and communicate with a neighbor. Instead, these amazing proteins facilitate communication between your cells

3   Enzymes which act like the electrical system of your home that causes many of your appliances to work. Enzymes provide the energy to spark changes in molecules and rebuild stress-damaged proteins.

**Figure 3** illustrates how LII's Anti-Aging Plan works by keeping the rate of cell repair and renewal greater than the rate of cell degeneration caused by stress and other environmental factors.

There is another reason why eating the correct forms of protein in our diet and supplements can stop the wear and tear of stress on our genes. During a stress reaction or emotional upheaval, hormones are thrown out of balance. In the rest of this book we will clearly explain

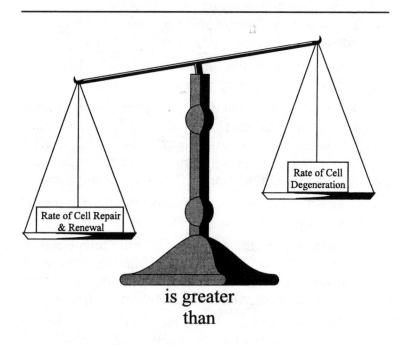

is greater
than

**Figure 3.** Slowing the age process means keeping the rate of cell repair and renewal greater than the rate of cell degradation.

the importance of eating the right type and balance of protein to slow down and even stop the wear and tear of everyday stress.

## ACCELERATED GUT AGING

Stress can weaken the digestive system and damage health. Research indicates that there are close relationships between stress, diet, and the digestive system that can influence the rate of aging in the body. Every time we have a stress reaction, the body diverts blood circulation away from the digestive tract to the heart and nervous system. Reduced circulation to the gut has a slow and insidious effect, greatly lessening the power of natural resistance to age-related diseases. And, this problem is only compounded when our diets are nutrient-poor to begin with.

Digestion is the chemical and physical process that the body uses to extract critical nutrients that we need for stress defense and for regeneration. If we are unable to assimilate these essential nutrients rapidly and efficiently, we will age faster than we should.

Each part of the digestive system needs to be in prime working order, or we age prematurely. The integrity of the digestive system itself relies on a sufficient store of appropriate stomach acid levels, liver-produced bile, and enzymes to break down foods into nutrients and then transport them throughout the body to where they are needed. When we are under stress, enzymes and other nutrients are used more quickly and so they continually need to be supplemented in our daily diets.

Authorities now are confident that maldigestion and malnourishment are the insidious precursors to most age-related diseases and dysfunctions.[2-9] The U.S. Center for Disease Control has concluded that antibiotics added to animal stock feed has caused animals to develop highly resistant strains of bacteria which are then passed on for human consumption, causing gut-related bacterial disorders in many people.[10] To make matters worse, we regularly consume over 10,000 food additives, pesticides and air pollutants that deplete nutrients. This causes the digestive system to become increasingly inefficient.[6,11,12]

In order to avoid the deleterious effects of stress, a program of highly specific foods and supplements, designed to unleash the body's own rejuvenative mechanisms of cell repair and renewal, is recommended. The LII Anti-Aging Plan provides a unique and patented nutritional supplementation program of bio-available nutrients and hormone precursors that result in the rapid and efficient absorption of nutrients into the cells—no matter how weak your digestive system may be. These supplements help the body coordinate trillions of cellular functions and reinforce the neuro-hormonal pathways.

Unlike other supplements currently available, these nutrients are energized with specific cellular electromagnetic resonances to speed up the process of cellular regeneration. These unique energies are programmed into special nutrient complexes to "switch on" anti-aging hormonal pathways and "switch off" the aberrant biochemical and hormonal pathways which are activated during the stress response. You will understand more about these super-charged nutrient complexes as you explore Chapter 6.

The Bottom Line: The faster we absorb and assimilate nutrients into our cells, the more HGH, IGF-1, and other anti-aging hormones we produce.

The Result: the slower we age.

## PREVENTING DIET-INDUCED STRESS DISORDERS

Every morning John prepares to start his day by exercising and eating a healthy breakfast. His breakfast: soybeans made with steel cut oats, turmeric, and other herbs. For lunch, he eats a spinach salad and lentil soup. When he gets home from work, his wife has a delicious dinner waiting for him: an appetizer of smoked salmon with horseradish, soup with tofu (bean curd), steamed bamboo shoots, cracked rye berries, and herbal tea.

John's twin sister Tara lives with her husband Mike who prefers to eat popular American foods. Tara and Mike typically eat bacon and eggs for breakfast, a fast food hamburger, slice of pizza or hoagie for lunch, followed later by meat and potatoes for dinner.

Both John and Tara are 45 years old. Despite a common gene pool, the truth is John looks about 15 years younger than Tara. John, it turns out, has a low risk of developing age-related illnesses, while Tara, on the other hand, is already suffering from numerous complex, age-related disorders.

This is because Tara has chosen the average American diet which averages about 40 percent fat, what is eight times the fat content of John's diet. Tara's diet is high in animal protein while John's diet is high in plant-based protein/carbohydrate combinations.

Manipulation of the diet is a vital factor in preventing age-related diseases. Foods fall into two general categories—those that have been linked to accelerated aging (age-accelerating foods) and those that offer protection against it (age-reversing foods).

Here's a partial list of age-accelerating versus age-reversing foods:

| Age-Accelerators | Age-Reversing Foods |
| --- | --- |
| Frankfurters | Broccoli |
| Bacon | Spinach |
| Sausage | Brussels sprouts |
| Bologna | Cabbage |
| Luncheon meats | Tomatoes |
| Butter | Green leafy vegetables |
| Cream and Sour Cream | Root vegetables |
| Cream Cheese | Lettuce |
| Margarine | Sprouts |
| Mayonnaise | Steel-cut Oats |
| Sugar | Lentils |
| Refined Flours | Legumes |
| Saccharin | String beans |
| Coffee | Fish |
| Alcoholic Beverages | Sunflower seeds |
| Pork | Almonds (raw) |
| Meats | Wheat Germ |
| | Macadamia nuts |

If your diet is high in *age-accelerator* foods and low in *age-reversing* foods, you may want to rethink your diet. Mounting evidence indicates that what you eat greatly affects your rate of aging. Focusing on age reversing foods while cutting down on *age-accelerator* foods will also help to reduce the level of diet-induced stress and enhance the function of your digestive tract. By eliminating or reducing the foods that place us at risk for age-related diseases, we have a high level of individual control over stress.

You will learn more about the importance of diet in balancing hormones, boosting anti-aging pathways of the body, and improving digestive function when you study Chapter 9. It is so simple!

## POINTS TO REMEMBER...

♦ Stress-induced wear and tear of our genetic blueprints can be prevented and even reversed.

♦ Recognizing stress in your life is the first step toward defending your body from the ravages of stress.

♦ Stress symptoms are actually early warning signals telling us that our lifestyle needs to be changed.

♦ Stress depletes protein and other nutrients the body needs to manufacture anti-aging hormones like HGH and IGF-1.

♦ Accelerated molecular and tissue aging involves stress-induced chemical and hormonal reactions that speed up our aging clocks and injure the DNA of our individual cells.

♦ Imbalances in our cellular soup lead to cell dysfunction and abnormalities in protein synthesis which slow down the repair and rebuilding functions of the body's genes.

## WHAT YOU CAN DO NOW

♦ Accept that stress is a part of life and that not all stress is bad.

♦ When in a stressful situation, take a series of deep breaths, stop and analyze the situation, and instead focus on a beach, sunset, or some other environment where you really become relaxed.

- ◆ Decrease your intake of *age-accelerating foods* to preserve and maintain your gene-activated stress repair mechanisms.

- ◆ Increase your intake of *age-reversing foods* which provide your body with the raw materials needed by your cellular soup to repair stress-induced damage.

- ◆ Get enough sleep. People who get enough rest do cope with stress better.

- ◆ Practice time management to reduce feelings of uncertainty and lack of control.

- ◆ Think of stress as the tension on guitar strings. Too much tension will make the guitar strings break. But, the right amount of tension produces beautiful music!

- ◆ Find time to relax and exercise. Concentrate on exploring Chapter 10, which gives valuable additional advice on stress reduction and exercise.

# CHAPTER 4

# THE LII ANTIOXIDANT DEFENSE PLAN

The body and its cells are damaged by biochemical compounds called free radicals. These compounds are highly reactive and toxic to the body's cells and DNA. Free radicals are generated by the breakdown of oxygen in the body causing damage to the tiny energy factories of the cell, called mitochondria. A free radical can be best described as an unstable oxygen molecule that possesses an unpaired electron. This molecule is constantly trying to become whole by robbing cells of vital components.

The body becomes more vulnerable to free radical damage with advancing age.

Free radicals actually burn holes in the cellular membranes in order to penetrate the inside of the body's cells. These tiny destroyers react rapidly with anything in their path, unleashing a destructive cascade of multiplying chemical reactions on our DNA and other vital cellular components. How can the body protect itself against the domino effect of free radical chain reactions? By means of powerful antioxidant nutrients in the body's cellular soup. These innate defenses consist of a select group of enzymes and nutrients that keep free radicals stable—stopping the domino effect or cascade of multiplying reactions.

Scientists now believe that free radical-induced damage to hormone receptors, enzymes, proteins, DNA, and cell membranes leads to the development of age-related diseases.[1-18]

## ANTIOXIDANT DEFENSES AND OXIDATION

Antioxidants can be defined as "fighters of oxygen." But why would we want to fight this life-sustaining element? The oxygen we breathe reacts with the body's chemicals to give us energy. Ninety-eight percent of the oxygen we breathe is combined with sugar and fats by the tiny energy-producing factories inside our cells called mitochondria. Oxygen's ability to combine with other chemicals, releasing energy in the process, is called oxidation.

A small number of oxygen molecules we breathe however, are converted into free radicals. Hence, some oxidation is unwanted and toxic to our cellular soup. Just as metals rust and a sliced apple turns brown from oxidation, fats in cell membranes can turn rancid and toxic with unwanted oxidation. Antioxidant nutrients act as protective substances to keep unwanted oxidation reactions under control. **Figure 4** illustrates how antioxidant nutrients in our cellular soup protect the cell by blocking unwanted oxidative damage to hormone receptors, the mitochondria, DNA, and other cellular components.

It is important to remember that not all free radical reactions are bad. In fact, the phagocyte cells of the immune system generate free radicals in the process of destroying invading bacteria, viruses, and other infectious organisms. Yet, these tiny renegades can become very destructive if they are not controlled with antioxidants. When the body lacks the right amounts of antioxidants, free radicals overpopulate the body causing premature aging and serious damage to the body.

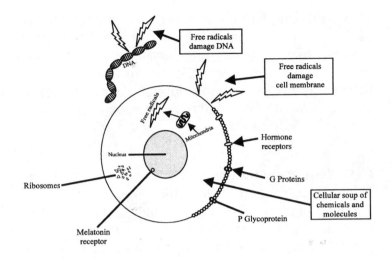

**Figure 4.** Illustration of how free radicals can damage hormone receptors and DNA. Antioxidants in our cellular soup shield the cellular world from free radicals.

In *The Antioxidants*, Richard Passwater, Ph.D.[4] outlines four basic ways that free radicals lead to damage and degeneration of the body:

**Lipid peroxidation**. Fats become rancid when they are attacked by free radicals. Since many forms of fats are involved in hormone transport and reception at the cellular membrane, it is easy to understand how lipid peroxidation reduces the activity of anti-aging hormones in the body.

41

**Cross-linking**. Hormones and many internal structures of the cell are made up of proteins. Free radicals alter the structure of proteins, causing them to fuse together. Once protein molecules are damaged in this manner, they lose their ability to function in a normal and natural manner. Most commonly, HGH and IGF-1 are damaged from what is called cross-linking.

**Cell Membrane Damage**. The cell membrane functions like a protective barrier and multi-operator switchboard, allowing certain substances to enter and exit the cell's internal world. Free radicals can punch holes in this protective barrier, thereby impairing the cell's ability to react appropriately to hormonal messengers, absorb nutrients and eliminate waste products.

**Lysosome Damage**. Deep within the cellular world are powerful digestive enzymes called lysosomes. By punching holes in the cell membrane, free radicals allow these important enzymes to escape and induce damage to the cell's outer environment (the extracellular matrix).

With an understanding of how free radicals contribute to the aging process, it is easier to see how they can lead to serious, life-threatening diseases.[5-9] Current research documents very clearly state that antioxidant nutrients and an antioxidant-rich diet will reduce your risk for the following age-related disorders:

*Alzheimer's disease* - by fortifying and supplying protective nutrients to the brain and nervous system and stopping the accumulation of damaged protein (amyloid) deposits;

*Diabetes* - by protecting the insulin-producing beta cells of the pancreas against oxidative damage;

*Arthritis* - by keeping immune defenses healthy and activating liver detoxification functions;

*Cardiovascular Diseases* - by preventing the oxidation of fats and low-density lipoproteins (LDLs)--a bad form of cholesterol that accumulates as plaque in the blood vessels;

*Hearing and Visual Disorders* - by reducing oxidative and accumulation of plaque in the tiny circulatory networks of the ear and eye.[19,20]

## WHAT CAUSES FREE RADICAL REACTIONS?

Shielding our cells from free radical bombardment protects us from injury-causing free radicals. Knowledge about the various causes of free radical reactions helps reduce the risk of excessive free-radical formation. The following external pollutants and biochemical processes of the body cause excessive free radical reactions:

**Environmental pollutants**. Today's world is full of toxins that we either breathe or ingest into our bodies. Many of these toxins either contain free radicals themselves or stimulate the production of free radicals after they enter our bodies. Nitrogen dioxide and nitrogen oxide in polluted air, cigarette smoke, radon gases, ozone, and automobile exhaust are examples of some of the free-radical generating toxins in the air we breathe. Radiation, pesticides, and chemicals are some examples of the free-radical generating toxins in our food supply.

**Appendix A** of this book lists those food additives that have known age-accelerating effects. Start to make note of these toxic chemicals, looking for them in the ingredients of the food you purchase.

**Stress**. As discussed in the previous chapter, stress is a cause of many age-related diseases. The almost infinite varieties of stress symptoms, from recurring headaches, ulcers, to high blood pressure, no matter how mild or severe, all increase the production of free radicals in the body. Whether stress causes high blood pressure that diminishes activity or crippling arthritis, the emotional component of the illness often accelerates the damages caused by stress. For example, the secretary with a headache, under pressure to produce work, suffers the stress of her headache plus the distress and fear of not being able to keep up with her job responsibilities.

If you are already ill or have numerous stress symptoms, your "emotional" stress levels may be far greater than a healthy person under the same stress conditions.

Trying to block the emotional symptoms of your illness with anti-anxiety or anti-depressive medication also increases the unwanted and excessive production of free radicals. While these medications may be necessary to relieve symptoms, they are not helpful over the long haul. It is important to keep in mind that most categories of illness, from mild to severe, share the same powerful effects of illness on the emotions and mind.

The need to deal with mind and emotions as well as physical problems is part and parcel of the LII Anti-Aging Plan. The mind is a powerful healer of the body. Self-help and awareness techniques can be far more powerful than drugs in the management of stress-induced illnesses.

At LII, we believe that patient education is an important part of our anti-aging plan. Chapter 8 provides helpful suggestions on how you can modify your lifestyle to get the full benefits of the LII Anti-Aging Plan. Understanding why and how we age allows the mind to focus on positive solutions.

**Antioxidant and Hormonal Deficiencies**. Even though free radicals occur as normal by-products of metabolism and the body's healthy response to stressors, they get "out of control" when we are deficient in antioxidants and hormones. A continuous battle is waged between free radicals and antioxidants (nutrients and some hormones) everyday in our bodies. With increasing levels of pollution and the fast-paced lifestyle of our American society, we need to build up our natural defense mechanisms against free radicals. If we fail to fortify our cellular soup with the essential biological weapons— adequate levels of nutrients, hormone precursors, and hormones—we age prematurely and free radicals wreck havoc in many vital aspects of body functioning, including our immune, cardiovascular, endocrine, and neurological systems.

We must continually strive to keep free radicals under control. The LII Anti-Aging Plan utilizes antioxidant and free radical scavengers designed to counteract and minimize the damaging effects of these compounds. This plan is designed to help you attain a prolonged, healthy, functional life and reduce your risk for the disease of aging.

Appropriate dietary intervention is an important part of the LII Anti-Aging Plan. Foods that are low in antioxidants and high in food additives need to be eliminated or reduced to low levels of dietary intake.

While we may not always be able to reduce the free radical-generating effects of air pollution, we can make a diligent effort to reduce our dietary intake of harmful free radical-generating foods.

## AVOIDING FREE-RADICAL GENERATING FOODS

The foods that contribute to the excessive production of free radicals fall into four basic categories:

1    Foods that are high in chemical additives (see Appendix);

2    Foods that are high in acid-producing factors;

3    Foods that are high in refined starches and sugars;

4    Foods that are high in saturated and trans fats.

Since we have already discovered how foods high in chemical additives produce free radical reactions, it is important to develop a basic understanding of how acid-producing foods, starches and sugars, as well as saturated and trans fats also cause free radical excesses in the body.

Before we discuss these three very important factors, you will need a basic understanding of the word "balance" and how we go about achieving it. In order to help you understand the meaning of the word "balance", picture a tightrope walker who cancels the downward pull of gravity by continuous action from side to side. The continuous action of antioxidants against free radicals protects us from premature aging. The reciprocal actions of two opposing forces in the body, antioxidants and free radicals, extend from one extreme, then the other, as on a pendulum or seesaw. As **Figure 5** illustrates,

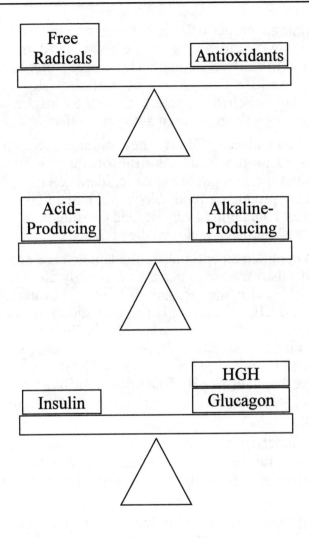

**Figure 5**. Maintaining the balance between free radicals/antioxidants, acid-producing/alkaline-producing, insulin/glucagon, and insulin/HgH ratios.

maintaining a proper balance between free radicals and antioxidants, acid and alkaline foods, and insulin (triggered in excessive amounts by simple starches and sugars) and glucagon (stimulated by the protein-fat-carbohydrate ratio), as well as insulin and HGH provides the maximum anti-aging effects.

**Acid-Producing Foods**. The continuous, reciprocal actions of acid versus alkaline-producing foods, determines the strength of our antioxidant defenses. Too many acid-producing foods block antioxidant enzymes and reduces our ability to digest food into micronutrients that nourish, protect, and revitalize our cells.

To maintain an optimal antioxidant defense against free radicals, we need to maintain a slightly alkaline or neutral pH. PH is the measure of how acid or alkaline you are. At LII, we assess pH and oxidation rates as an important part of our Biomarker Matrix Protocol™ for determining biological age. PH ranges from acid (4.5) to alkaline (8.0), with 7.0 being the neutral balance point. When we maintain the pH of our urine and saliva between 6.6 and 7.4, we excite powerful antioxidant activity in the body.

By understanding how your dietary choices govern the acid-alkaline balance in your body, you can work with, rather than against your natural antioxidant defense system.

In general, the following foods are acid-producing: sugar, white flour, most commercial cereals, fish, fowl, eggs, and meat. Alkaline-producing foods are fruits, all vegetables, legumes, and soy products. But, here is the important distinction: alkaline-producing foods have high antioxidant activity and acid-producing foods have virtually no antioxidant nutrients. Ideally, we need to consume 60 to 75 percent of alkaline-producing foods to keep our cellular soup in the pH range of high enzyme activity. Because stress and pollutants also acidify our bodies, maintaining the proper dietary ratio between acid-producing and alkaline-producing foods is an important part of the LII Anti-Aging Plan.

**Foods high in sugars and simple starches**. The food you eat has an exceptionally powerful effect of activating hormonal responses in the body. Eating too many sugars and simple carbohydrates depletes antioxidant nutrients and anti-aging hormones. Stripped of most of their naturally attendant nutrients, simple carbohydrates cannot be properly metabolized by the body. In fact, every time we eat them we amplify free radical activity, elevate stress-produced hormones, and create biochemical imbalances in the body.

The more processed food we consume, the more refined sugars and starches we consume. Simple carbohydrates are made up of short chains of sugars, causing the body to burn them quickly. On the other hand, complex carbohydrates (vegetables, legumes, whole grains) are made up of longer chains of sugars and proteins that are burned more slowly and efficiently by the body. **Figure 6** illustrates how sugar metabolism can be stabilized by consuming complex carbohydrates that have the correct amounts of protein and fats. The quick bursts of energy we get from sugars and simple carbohydrates cause our blood sugar and insulin levels to go up and down like a roller coaster. In comparison, the slow-released energy of complex carbohydrates keeps our hormones balanced and our energy levels stable. When our energy levels are steady and continuous, our antioxidant defenses exert constant pressure against free radicals—keeping them at levels that inhibit the aging process.

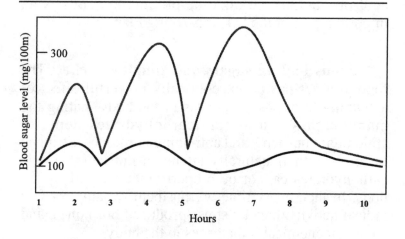

**Figure 6.** The roller coaster effect of simple sugars and carbohydrates vs the stable blood sugar of carbohydrates that are high in protein.

**Foods high in saturated and trans fats**. High levels of cholesterol, triglycerides, and LDL cholesterol are high risk factors that put you in the danger zone for cardiovascular diseases. The good news is that you can do a great deal to lower these dangerously high fats and elevate the "good" cholesterol (high-density lipoprotein). By cutting out or reducing your intake of animal fats and protein and at the same time increasing your intake of monosaturated fats like olive oil, you can lower LDL and elevate HDL to normal levels. By balancing these dietary fats at the correct levels, you reduce oxidation dramatically and improve hormone transport and activation in the body. Why is this so important?

Remember, oxidation causes fats to turn rancid. Excessive amounts of LDL cholesterol in your circulatory system is much like a traffic jam in your arteries. Oxidated LDL sticks to artery walls, reducing the delivery of life-sustaining, anti-aging nutrients to organ systems of the body. Trans fats, derived from processed, refined, or hydrogenated oils also clog arterial walls.

To illustrate what happens, picture a buildup of scale in your household plumbing. Your sluggish tap is caused by years of accumulation of minerals that stick to the inner linings of pipes, reducing the water flowing from your faucet. Although one solution would be to have a plumber replace all the pipes, the problem will only occur repeatedly until you reduce the amount of minerals in your water supply.

The same principle applies to the sludge or plaguing of your arteries. You can undergo a coronary artery bypass operation, in which a surgeon takes blood vessels, usually from your leg, to give your heart new arteries. However, if you do nothing to remove the cause of this arterial sludge, your "new" coronary arteries, too, will eventually become clogged.

**Table 1** illustrates desirable anti-aging and antioxidant levels for cholesterol, LDL cholesterol, HDL cholesterol, and triglycerides. Keeping your lipid levels within these ranges will help reduce your risk for arteriosclerosis and heart disease. Remember, LDL is oxidized by free radicals to cause hardening of the arteries. HDL, on the other hand, prevents the oxidation of LDL and even repairs free radical-damaged LDL.

As an added bonus, maintaining the proper levels of HDL enhances the body's ability to manufacture powerful anti-aging hormones like pregnenolone, DHEA, testosterone, and anti-inflammatory hormones like cortisone. You will discover even more about the hormonal connection to HDL and the aging process in the following chapter.

## TABLE 1 - IDEAL ANTIOXIDANT/ANTI-AGING LEVELS

| Measure | General Ranges | Antioxidant/Anti-aging Levels |
| --- | --- | --- |
| Cholesterol | <240 | <190 |
| LDL cholesterol | <160 | <130 |
| HDL cholesterol | >35 | >45 for men; >55 for women |
| Triglycerides | <250 | <150 |

## POINTS TO REMEMBER...

♦ The LII Anti-Aging Plan applies a comprehensive approach to reducing your risk for developing heart disease, stroke, and other diseases of the circulatory system.

♦ The LII Anti-Aging Plan provides full protection by fortifying your cellular soup against free radicals.

♦ Antioxidants protect your genetic blueprint against the free radical renegades that burn holes through cell membranes.

♦ By avoiding simple carbohydrates and sugars, you can maintain a healthy insulin/glucagon ratio, allowing your pituitary gland and liver to produce youthful levels of HGH and IGF-1.

## WHAT CAN YOU DO NOW

♦ Start by having your serum cholesterol, LDL cholesterol, HDL cholesterol, and triglycerides measured to determine if you are in the desirable range given in Table 1.

♦ If your test results are out of balance for the antioxidant and anti-aging desired levels, you will need to carefully read Chapter 8 and 9 for specific dietary and nutritional instructions developed to maximize your antioxidant and anti-aging levels of fat metabolism.

♦ Decrease your dietary intake of free-radical generating foods that are high in chemical additives, acid-producing factors, refined sugars, starches, and saturated as well as trans fats.

♦ Concentrate on Chapter 8 to learn about the LII-tested antioxidant nutritional formula.

♦ Concentrate on Chapter 9 to make your own grocery shopping list of foods high in antioxidants.

♦ Read through APPENDIX A for a list of age-accelerating food additives to avoid in your diet.

♦ Concentrate on Chapter 7 to find out about the specific details regarding the anti-aging and gene-protecting benefits of this plan.

# CHAPTER 5

# FINE-TUNING THE NEUROENDOCRINE ORCHESTRA

The neuroendocrine theory views the aging process as a decline in the ability of the nervous and endocrine systems to regulate and integrate the body's metabolic activities.

Neuroendocrine-produced hormones such as melatonin, as well as the other anti-aging hormones like hgh, igf-1, and dhea decline as much as 10 percent per decade. According to this theory, aging causes many endocrine glands to fatigue and become exhausted from overstimulation and overuse. When glands become weak and tired, their ability to respond quickly and effectively to the many stresses of life is diminished. For this reason, the saliva or blood levels of many endocrine-produced hormone levels are important biomarkers of the aging process.

Decreased hormonal secretions result in a body-wide imbalance that decreases the function of our immune system, metabolism, and sexual function. The profound effects of hormone replacement therapy on virtually all cells of the body provide a direct way to stimulate high levels of rejuvenative therapy to the body. As levels of these hormones are increased, the functional activity of many physiological processes are also enhanced.

## WHAT ARE HORMONES?

Hormones have a multitude of functions in the body. Some hormones function as chemical messengers that initiate, orchestrate, and influence the activity of body processes. Other hormones function as biological pacemakers that keep the body balanced.

Like the conductor of an orchestra, hormones attempt to maintain harmony and balance in the body. Hormones can <u>activate</u> or <u>deactivate</u> many functions of the body. **Figure 7** illustrates how hormones can be blocked by genetic damage and free radical degradation. The production, activity, transport, and reception of hormones can be hyperactive or underactive, causing many illnesses.

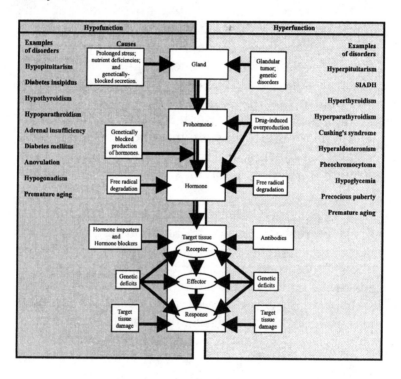

**Figure 7.** Causes of neuroendocrine dysfunction.

Hormones are classified into four types: peptides, steroids, amino acid analogues, and fatty acid derivatives. The peptides include hormones secreted by the pituitary gland (HGH), the parathyroids, and the pancreas. Insulin and glucagon secreted by the pancreas are examples of peptide hormones. The steroids are made from cholesterol and include hormones produced by the adrenal glands (DHEA, cortisol, cortisone, etc.) and the gonads (estrogen, testosterone). The amino acid analogues include the thyroid hormones and another group of hormones secreted by the adrenals called catecholamines (norepinephrine and epinephrine). Fatty acid derived hormones are the prostaglandins, more recently referred to as ecosanoid hormones.

Hormones travel to receptor sites, located on the cell membrane or inside the cellular environment. When they make contact with a receptor, they deliver a chemical message that changes the cell's behavior.

Hormones are produced from precursors, compounds, and enzymes by way of a step-by-step biochemical process. If only one enzyme or nutrient is missing in this biochemical process, the body may fail to produce the needed hormones. However, the decline in the body's production of many hormones with advancing age is related to an inability to digest, absorb, assimilate, or utilize one or more of the following precursors:

♦ hydrolyzed protein fragments known as bioactive peptides in order to facilitate the natural production of peptide hormones like HGH and IGF-1;

♦ amino acids (smallest units of digested protein) in order to facilitate the natural production of amino acid analogue hormones;

57

♦ fatty acids, fatty acid esters and HDL cholesterol in order to facilitate the natural production of steroid hormones like pregnenolone, DHEA, and testosterone.

**Figure 8** illustrates how enzyme deficits due to a weak digestive system can block the production of peptide and amino acid analogue hormones. Our research shows that individuals who age prematurely have weak gut functions that limit their ability to assimilate hormone precursors into the biochemical pathways of hormone production (**Figure 9**).

In the chapters that follow, you will learn what supplements and foods boost digestive capacity, allowing your body to rapidly absorb these vital precursors to make an abundant supply of anti-aging hormones. You will also learn the critical importance of HDL cholesterol as a carrier of many hormones. And, as previously discussed, we'll recommend a diet plan that keeps your LDL cholesterol less than 130 and your HDL cholesterol around 45 (women) and 55 (men). All this unique information translates into enhanced hormonal production, transport and a dramatic reduction of destructive free radicals.

## HORMONES AND PREMATURE AGING

Hormones effect aging in a multitude of ways. Premature aging of the endocrine glands affects skin, hair, body-fat composition, muscles and bones, and all organs of the body. Some hormones affect the secretion of products of the digestive tract, such as enzymes, hydrochloric acid, and bile salts; the synthesis and degradation of carbohydrates, lipids and proteins to meet specific energy needs of the individual. Hormones also

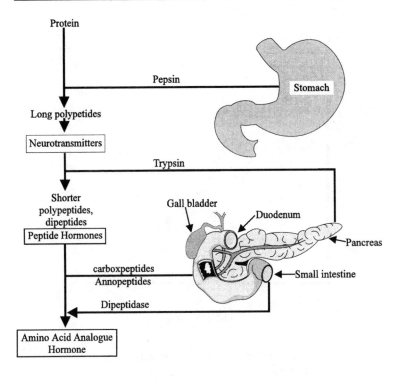

**Figure 8.** The transformation of protein into peptide hormones and amino acid analogue hormones via enzymatic actions of the gut.

affect contraction, relaxation, and metabolism of muscles, vascular and heart musculature, as well as the GI and genital tract musculature. As discussed previously, many functions regulated by hormones result from the interaction of the hormone with specific receptors.

Supplementation of hormones without understanding the cellular response to hormonal stimulation—determined by the health, pH and nutritional status of the receptor cell—causes many hormone

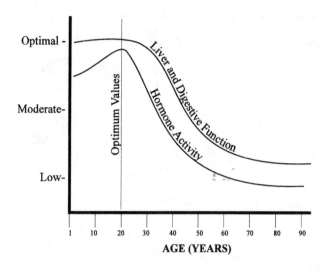

**Figure 9.** The reduction of hormonal, liver and digestive function with advancing age.

replacement therapies to have minimal anti-aging effects. If hormones cannot bind to appropriate receptor sites—they have no anti-aging effects.

Hormonal disorders are estimated to affect 40% of all American women between the age of 14 and 50 who suffer with Premenstrual Syndrome (PMS). Twelve percent of American women are severely debilitated with PMS. Functional weaknesses of the thyroid gland and adrenals affect over 50% of the population and are the leading cause of chronic fatigue, immune dysfunction, inflammatory and allergic conditions.

Doctors commonly prescribe thyroid hormone or cortisone for these disorders—even though they fail to strengthen and fortify these glands. As a result, endocrine glands continue to age and anti-aging hormone levels continue to decline in these individuals.

As explained previously, the stress from dietary errors produces profound neuroendocrine disturbances in the body. These disturbances diminish the biological integrity and erode the psychological potential of humans. The LII Anti-Aging Plan can counteract these reactions and provide a reliable and effective strategy for survival and the maintenance of well-being.

## THE NEUROENDOCRINE ORCHESTRA

Hormones work together, not in isolation from one another. Synergism exists between many hormones and the nervous system of the body. The nervous system and the endocrine system orchestrate the function of some 50 billion cells, a process we call the neuroendocrine orchestra (**Figure 10**).

The nervous system meets the endocrine system at the hypothalamic-pituitary interface. At this site, neural and hormonal pathways of communication regulate hundreds of chemical reactions involved in many functions of the body.

Hormones stimulate and regulate a multitude of life-giving processes throughout the body. Hormonal regulation patterns help to maintain health, harmony, growth, healing and repair.

The pituitary gland, known as the master gland, functions like the conductor of an orchestra, keeping all the body's hormones in balance. Just as a thermostat is

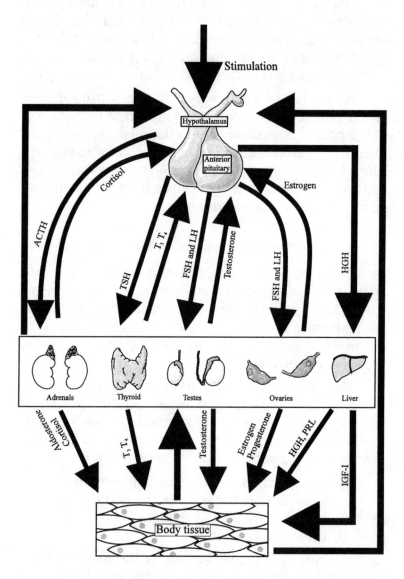

**Figure 10.** The Neuroendocrine Orchestra.

satisfied when the room temperature reaches the setting of the thermostat, the pituitary is satisfied when the hormone production of various glands are adequate.

When we are young and resilient, the feedback system between the hypothalamic-pituitary interface and other endocrine glands is under fixed and rigid control. But, with aging, this feedback system responds inefficiently to the needs of the body. In many cases, the pituitary gland overworks when it is unable to synchronize, or reestablish glandular relationships on a normal plane. Eventually, the pituitary gland reaches a point of exhaustion and our HGH and IGF-1 levels decline dramatically. At this point, the adrenal cortex tries to compensate by managing the gonads and to some extent the pancreas. However, this back-up plan of the neuroendocrine system has four major limitations:

1    The adrenal cortex is not capable of managing the thyroid gland constantly causing thyroid gland function to operate too fast or too slow. When the thyroid gland weakens from overuse, the hypothalamic area of the brain and pineal gland try to maintain balance of hormones.

2    Eventually, the pineal gland overworks and also tires out. The result: decreased levels of melatonin, epithalamin and other compounds produced by the pineal gland. Contrary to the popular belief, supplementing with "melatonin alone" does not address the full complexity of these issues of neuroendocrine dysregulation.

3    The functional decline of the pituitary gland continues to reduce HGH and IGF-1 levels causing many organs and organ systems to age and perform poorly and inefficiently.

4   Overstimulation of the adrenals activates a very destructive age-accelerating process: Protein is depleted from the liver and gut, leaving less protein available for the body to formulate needed HGH, IGF-1, and other critical hormones.

Although this process sounds complicated and hard to understand, it is important to understand how someone can enter a vicious cycle of aging that can not be compensated for by single hormone therapies.

LII's Anti-Aging Plan is superior to these "symptom-based," anti-aging hormone replacement therapies because we address the full complexity of all these related issues. Our objective: To get your entire neuroendocrine system balanced and functioning at peak capacity.

Again, just consider how the thermostat in your home works. The interrelationship of the pituitary gland with other endocrine (target) glands is maintained in a state of equilibrium when the target gland satisfies the demand for a given hormone. In this fashion, the pituitary acts like a thermostat that is satisfied when the heat level reaches the setting of the thermostat. When the heat level falls below the setting of the thermostat, the furnace is activated to produce more heat. When an endocrine (target) gland fails to produce its particular hormone, the pituitary gland, not being satisfied relentlessly continues to stimulate the sluggish target gland. Eventually, the pituitary gland gets tired and is unable to synchronize, or balance hormones. However, the body has an "emergency back-up plan:" the hypothalamic area of the brain takes part of the effort into the pineal gland for the release of melatonin during sleep cycles of the body. But as these back-up patterns of physiology continue, we eventually deplete and exhaust the pineal gland.

Women who have had hysterectomies function in these back-up neuroendocrine pathways because the pituitary gland is unable to influence ovaries that are no longer present. For long periods of time, the pituitary gland will overwork trying to excite the production of ovarian-produced hormones. When HDL cholesterol is too low and LDL cholesterol is too high, there is double trouble in these cases. Normally, the adrenals will produce DHEA which can be converted to ovarian hormones to satisfy the pituitary's demand for balanced levels of these hormones. In these cases, our research has shown that supplementation with Pregnenolone (PREG) and DHEA help to compensate for the surgical removal of the ovaries. You will learn more about how the body can make sex hormones from PREG and DHEA later in this chapter.

LII scientists and other anti-aging medical experts believe that hormonal imbalances are not understood by the isolated treatment of one gland. The main focus of this field of medicine is on the prevention of age-related diseases. Individuals who complain of chronic fatigue, various states of exhaustion and maldigestion are suffering from an imbalance of the entire neuroendocrine system, not just a single gland dysfunction.

Like a beautiful symphony produced by talented musicians, the neuroendocrine orchestra is a symphony only when all hormone-producing glands function properly and harmonize with other systems of the body in a synchronized manner. The entire "neuroendocrine" symphony may be one harsh discordant noise when physicians treat only one gland or prescribe merely an isolated hormone.

This Anti-Aging Plan is designed to untangle the complex myriad of neuroendocrine symptoms so that rejuvenation of the aging body is optimal.

Ulcers, hepatitis, gallstones, gastritis, colitis, pancreatitis, diverticulitis, yeast and fungal infections of the GI system, cancers of the colon, pancreas, stomach, liver and esophagus all involve hormone deficits and imbalances. Early and commonly neglected digestive symptoms (indigestion, heartburn, vomiting, abdominal discomfort and pain, flatulence, constipation, and diarrhea) are biomarkers of the aging process. Yet, over 50% of Americans complain of the frequent occurrence of these common symptoms, purchasing over-the-counter remedies for these complaints.

Covering up these early signs of premature aging only serves to accelerate the aging process. Instead, the LII Anti-Aging Plan helps individuals understand the underlying causes of these symptoms. Rather than treat the symptoms while aging accelerates, the LII Anti-Aging Plan addresses the genetic and molecular causes of premature aging. The goal: to emphasize prevention by teaching individuals the components of a healthy lifestyle.

Scientists at LII have come to the realization that most "official" medical ills give neuroendocrine signals long before a breakdown of bodily parts occurs. All illness has an incubation period, the time it takes before some physical or emotional distress becomes disturbing enough to be traditionally diagnosed. Some diseases, such as the wear and tear problems that lead to glandular exhaustion, can incubate into cancer with only vague and ambiguous signs for years. During their incubation period, physical and emotional symptoms alter normal body physiology and produce neuroendocrine changes that cannot be detected and documented by standard medical tests. These signs and signals that foreshadow a disease of the aging process can readily be observed with the LII

Biomarker Matrix Protocol™ long before the ailment becomes irreversibly serious and damaging.

Compared to many animals, mankind has the most highly developed and dynamic of all neuroendocrine systems. A symptom or set of symptoms is merely the expression of hormonal imbalances or faulty hormonal reception and transmission. Modern Medicine in its preoccupation with chasing, labeling or diagnosing symptoms, has neglected the body's ability to orchestrate powerful anti-aging hormone responses!

The neuroendocrine orchestra is continually related to the many other subsystems of the body in an interactive network of reciprocal relationships. Taking too much of any single hormone may disturb these interactive networks. Seen in this light, illness is the result of a disturbance in the orchestration of the entire neuroendocrine response within the body's interactive structures—with no one hormone or substance being able to correct the totality of disturbances in the overall human organism.

For the first time, the LII Anti-Aging Plan addresses malfunctions in the orchestration or the transmission and processions of information in these intermeshed neuroendocrine networks to slow down accelerated aging at many levels simultaneously.

The LII Anti-Aging Plan and the Biomarker Matrix Protocol™ employ a comprehensive approach to fine-tuning the neuroendocrine orchestra. Organizing and restoring control of these biological functions results in normal neuroendocrine regulation, producing an age-reversal effect that far surpasses "single hormone" replacement therapies.

In spite of some impressive clinical results with hormone replacement therapy, supplementing hormones has not yet been demonstrated to convincingly increase the human life span. The primary reason for the apparent lack of effectiveness relates to how the endocrine system makes, transports, and reacts to signal-bearing hormones.

## Hormone Action, Transport And Reception

Hormones communicate with various parts of the body at the endocrine, paracrine, autocrine, and intracrine levels (**Figure 11**). At the endocrine level, hormones are secreted by special glands for release into the general circulation and transport to distant target cells. At the paracrine level, hormones released from one cell can influence neighboring cells. At the autocrine level, hormones secreted by a cell can exert positive or negative action to the same cell. At the intracrine level, hormones are formed and do not have to be released outside the cell membranes to change the function of the cell.[1-9]

When hormones are balanced at all four levels of hormone activity, the body automatically balances itself after a stressful event. The neuroendocrine orchestra regulates quickly and economically. In other words, the regulation of hormones occurs at the shortest route and in the least amount of time with a minimal expenditure of energy. Balanced hormonal activity means that your body can cope with stressors in a flexible, incredibly fast and dynamic manner according to the strength of the stress factor. This sensitive, delicately balanced, system of stress defense can be thrown out of balance by taking too many hormones or by eating the wrong foods.

When we age prematurely, the endocrine system becomes less responsive to external messages. Since

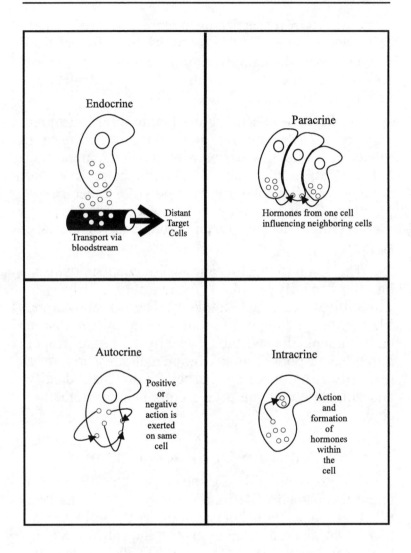

**Figure 11.** Levels of Hormone Activity.

hormones act by first attaching to a receptor on their target cells, the decline of these receptors from free radical damage can block or impede hormone activity. The aging endocrine system responds with rigid, slow, and inflexible activity to the stresses of life.

As **Figure 12** illustrates, maintaining hormone activity at the endocrine, paracrine, autocrine, and intracrine levels provides us with maximum anti-aging effects. Unlike other methods of hormone replacement therapy, the LII Anti-Aging Plan provides a therapeutic program that augments hormone production, transmission, and reception on all four levels of hormone activity.

The youthful, healthy and well-regulated organism has the capacity to adapt to the stress of life with extraordinary ease and simplicity. The LII Anti-Aging Plan improves an individual's adaptability to the environment, that is, their capacity to evoke proper hormonal responses to environmental stressors. As a result, the LII Anti-Aging Plan helps individuals identify and eliminate the causative factors behind premature aging.

## THE FORMATION OF STEROID HORMONES

Pregnenolone (PREG), known since the 1940's is a direct precursor to DHEA and many other hormones. PREG is made from cholesterol under the influence of thyroid hormone by way of an enzyme called Lecithin Cholesterol Acetyl Transferase (LCAT). PREG sits at the top of the biochemical pathway of every steroid hormone (**Figure 13**). Another enzyme, Cytochrome P450, involved in detoxification processes of the liver, assists in the conversion of PREG to other hormones. An

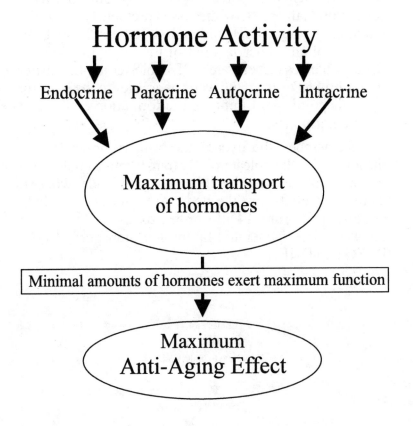

**Figure 12.** Maintaining hormone activity at the endocrine, paracrine, autocrine, and intracrine levels.

impairment of LCAT or P450 enzymes, common with premature aging, results in a blockage of the biochemical pathways of PREG.

Because the liver produces bile which emulsifies cholesterol into cholesterol esters and HDL cholesterol is the carrier of cholesterol, a healthy liver is necessary for the efficient transport of cholesterol to sites of PREG formation in the cells. As discussed previously, naturally enhancing your HGH and IGF-1 levels clears LDL cholesterol and other fats out of the body. In addition, dietary changes that elevate HDL cholesterol—the carrier of harmful LDL from the walls of arteries to the liver for rapid disposal—can improve the formation of all your steroid hormones.

Remember, the liver is the primary organ for the disposal of LDL cholesterol. By transforming cholesterol into bile salts or excreting it into the gallbladder where it can be excreted from the body. Antioxidants also help because as **Figure 14** illustrates, oxidative stress can block the liver-generated lipoprotein transport of both PREG and DHEA.

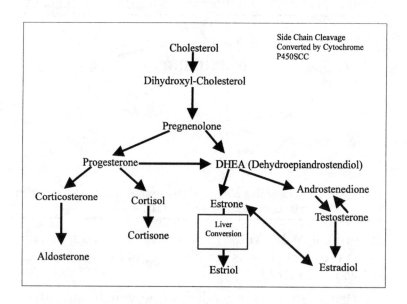

**Figure 13.** The Biochemical Pathways of Pregnenolone.

Our research has shown that the majority of individuals with low levels of PREG, DHEA, progesterone, estrogen, or testosterone have functional disorders of the liver. By assessing oxidative stress and pH, the Biomarker Matrix Protocol™ helps to predict the detoxification functions of the liver.

In addition, functional liver tests that challenge the liver detoxification networks document that many individuals have deficiencies of the P450 enzymes. In addition, in the process of being converted to DHEA and sex hormones, both PREG and DHEA go through chemical processes called conjugation and sulfation, another way the liver detoxifies the body. When P450 enzymes are impaired and chemical detoxification functions (conjugation and sulfation) are inadequate, the biochemical pathways of hormone formation fail to produce the quantity and quality of hormones necessary to counteract the aging process.

## POINTS TO REMEMBER...

The formation of hormones is dependent on the following:

♦ A healthy genetic blueprint and an ample supply of anti-aging nutrients in our cellular soup.

♦ Oxidative stress is reduced in the liver by improving enzymatic and chemical detoxification functions and by maintaining the proper balance between antioxidants and free radicals.

♦ The enzyme activity of our cellular soup— governed by pH and maintained by a proper acid/

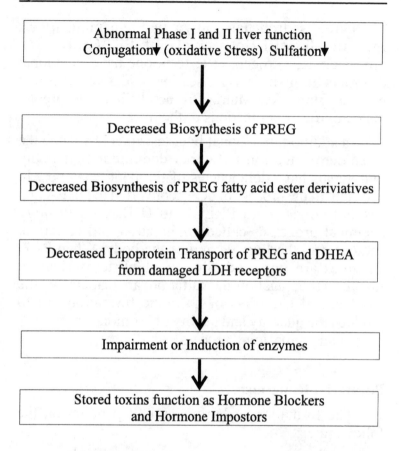

**Figure 14.** Lipoprotein Transport of PREG and DHEA,
altered by oxidative stress of the liver.

alkaline dietary balance—determines the
efficiency of many anti-aging mechanisms in the
body.

♦ Maintaining the proper levels of total cholesterol,
LDL cholesterol, HDL cholesterol, and

74

triglycerides by consuming less saturated fats but more monosaturated fats.

♦ Excessive or diminished hormone secretions cause most age-related disorders.

♦ Boosting HGH and IGF-1 concentrations that cause us to burn fat and build muscle mass naturally and increase all functions of the body.

Also, please keep in mind the following:

♦ Taking too much of a single hormone will disturb the delicate balance of the neuroendocrine system.

♦ Hormone Replacement Therapy is only effective when medically monitored and doses are tailored to meet the individual's needs.

♦ The LII Anti-Aging Plan is designed to properly balance the body's hormones on the endocrine, paracrine, autocrine, and intracrine levels, thus providing it with maximum anti-aging effects that maintain the integrity of each individual's genetic blueprint.

## WHAT YOU CAN DO NOW

♦ Don't take excessive amounts of vitamins or hormones without proper medical supervision by an LII-trained physician.

♦ Concentrate on eating less refined sugars and starches to maintain your insulin/glucagon ratio.

♦ Concentrate on reducing your saturated fat levels to maintain the activity and transport of your hormones.

♦   Read and pay special attention to the following two chapters which provide you with valuable recommendations on hormone precursors called secretagogues and the nutritional factors that will fine-tune your neuroendocrine system and boost your levels of HGH and IGF-1.

# CHAPTER 6

# HGH, IGF-1 AND OTHER MIRACLE HORMONES

HGH and IGF-1 have astounding age-reversal effects that promise to be powerful weapons against age-related diseases. They have the amazing ability to restore biological vigor and balance in the neuroendocrine system. The age-related decline in the production of these amazing hormones is related to a depleted molecular and chemical status within our cellular soup.

When we keep our cellular soup alive and nutrient-dense, we activate cells of the pituitary gland to produce youthful levels of HGH. Rather than accept abdominal bulging, the wrinkling of our skin, and the flabbiness of our muscles as the inevitable consequence of a HGH decline, we can enhance the production of HGH and IGF-1 with the LII Anti-Aging Plan.

## INSULIN AND HGH

With advancing age, we lose the ability to metabolize glucose effectively. We become less sensitive to the actions of insulin. And, in many cases, insulin malfunctions by converting glucose into fat cells. When we elevate HGH, we redirect the action of insulin to inject the glucose into our cellular soup rather than fat cells, where it can energize and ignite a multitude of cellular functions.

Although HGH works by keeping insulin stable when stress or our diets provoke the release of excessive insulin, the ratios of insulin and glucagon are primarily controlled by our food choices.

The ability of the body to maintain the proper balance between insulin and glucagon declines with age. For over 70 years researchers have found that blood levels of insulin increase sharply as we age.[1,2] The body's ability to utilize glucose—a fundamental source of energy for the formation of hormones—is controlled by the insulin/glucagon ratio. Thyroid hormones also play a role in maintaining blood sugar levels.

Now, let's look at what happens when HGH concentrations remain lower than insulin. When insulin stays at high concentrations for too long a period of time, it creates fat (lipogenesis). As HGH declines, the body becomes more and more sensitive to sugars and simple carbohydrates.

How does the body react? High insulin levels flood our bodies with short bursts of excessive glucose followed by rapid drops in glucose. The result: We crave more sugar or addictive chemicals like caffeine and we enter the vicious cycle of accelerated aging.

Simple carbohydrates, sugars, alcohol, and caffeine overstimulate the production of insulin. These dietary factors also trigger a stress response, elevating stress hormones and depleting DHEA and other anti-aging hormones. The body responds to these blood sugar and insulin surges by altering the function of a whole array of internal processes (circulation, respiration, digestion, etc.).

That's why the dietary foundation for achieving a balance between insulin, glucagon, and HGH includes a daily intake of biologically-active proteins, called secretagogues.

You'll find more vital information about secretagogues and how to maintain the proper balance of insulin, glucagon, and HGH in Chapters 8 and 9.

It has been determined that natural substances, functioning as precursors of hormones can provide superior ways to stimulate regulation and regeneration of the neuroendocrine orchestra. This new insight directs us toward the humble recognition that natural and organic whole food complexes, hormones and hormone precursors can evoke powerful healing responses— thereby regenerating the body and slowing down the aging process.

## HGH, IGF-1 AND THE CELLULAR SOUP

As discussed previously, HGH is a small peptide-like hormone that is converted by the liver into IGF-1. Studies have shown that HGH production declines after the age of 20 at the rate of 14 percent per decade. By 60 years of age, it is not uncommon to measure a HGH loss of 75 percent or more. What, exactly, can HGH do to protect and preserve our genetic blueprint?

Let us give you a "nutshell" overview of the potential HGH and IGF-1 have in keeping your body in tip-top shape—intelligence, memory, as well as all of your physical functions:

- ◆ They control all regulation, regeneration and cell replacement in the body.

- ◆ They treat the genetic blueprint by initiating the transport of proteins and nucleic acids into our cellular soup giving DNA the raw material it needs to repair itself better.

79

◆ They promote the production of DNA, RNA, and proteins causing an increase in cell size and rate of cell division.

◆ They optimize all cellular and organ functions by turning old cells into new ones.

◆ They put the brakes on insulin, keeping our energy levels optimal, even when we go off our diets.

But, that's just part of the HGH and IGF-1 story. We know that people who have normal values of these hormones are active in their seventies, eighties, and nineties. They're traveling, playing golf, and living active and fulfilling lives.

## THE LIVER'S ROLE: HGH AND IGF-1

Here's another important consideration: Boosting our levels of IGF-1 depends on the liver's ability to convert HGH to IGF-1. Hence, the most important consideration in getting both these hormones to anti-aging levels, is the functional and nutritional status of the liver.

Our clinical studies have shown that many individuals who suffer from chronic headaches have a deficit in liver-related protein metabolism which causes the pituitary gland to overwork and expand. Deficits in the function of insulin render the liver unable to supply necessary blood sugar. Stress-induced adrenal cortical activity and an insulin/glucagon imbalance cause the liver to make glucose out of protein (gluconeogenesis) in a last ditch of effort to regulate blood sugar. As a result, HGH replacement therapy without knowledge of the intricate web of interdependent, overlapping and complex functions of other systems of the body may be in vain—

with no anti-aging effects. But, for the most part, clinical results with HGH replacement therapy appear quite promising.

There is powerful synergism between HGH and other hormones. Previously, we discussed how HGH and IGF-1 initiate the transport of proteins into the cell to facilitate the repair of cellular structures and genetic materials in our cellular soup. These two hormones are rapid accelerators of numerous repair and regenerative mechanisms in the body and have the most powerful anti-aging effect of all hormones. Furthermore, they stop aging at the most fundamental level of life—the cell.

A great deal of aging takes place at the cellular level because of a breakdown in the production of proteins (protein synthesis). This breakdown in protein synthesis is caused by a reduction in digestive capacity and liver function with advancing age and free radical attacks that damage and degrade proteins in the body's cells.

By increasing our levels of HGH we halt gluconeogenesis and prevent the liver from becoming debilitated and unable to remove or to inactivate excessive amounts of hormones. Improved androgen or estrogen levels are also the amazing result of this therapy.

Gluconeogenesis causes a lack of protein in the liver and an inadequate production level of a protein called albumin. Depressed levels of albumin are associated with fluid retention or edema in many individuals. Fluid retention is also caused by excessive stress which weakens the many diverse hormonal deactivating or activating functions of the liver. Thus, improving the health of the liver is necessary for the proper conversion of HGH and other hormones that keep the aging process in check.

By means of the chemical activity known as oxidation, reduction, and conjugation, the liver assists in the regulation and synchronization of the entire hormonal system.

The liver uses oxygen to neutralize the excessive amounts of hormones produced in response to the stresses of life, inactivating those hormones by forming salts and removing oxygen. This process is known as reduction. In addition, the liver uses another method called conjugation to join or bind excessive amounts of hormones together in order to restrict their activity. Researchers at LII have been studying the relationship between pH, oxidation and reduction in the liver as they relate to the activity or inactivity of hormones. To date, we have found the liver to have functional deficits in regulating hormones in the majority individuals.

It is common to find the liver debilitated and low in protein. When this happens the body resorts to cannibalistic utilization of protein from the gut, nervous system and liver.

Since storage of protein is very meager in the nervous system, it requires very little depletion of protein to precipitate neuritis, neuralgia's, nervous exhaustion or nervous breakdown. Other age-related conditions such as arthritis, hypertension, gastric and duodenal ulcers, arteriosclerosis and skeletal muscle spasms are also caused by disorders of protein synthesis.

HGH and IGF-1 serve the important function of increasing protein synthesis, thus preventing the cannibalistic utilization of protein from the gut, nervous system and liver, a major cause of the aging process.

HGH replacement therapy (by Daniel Rudman, M.D. of the Medical College of Wisconsin) has resulted in groundbreaking clinical results. In his study, twenty-one men between the ages of 61 and 81 received HGH injections. The results demonstrated a ten to twenty year reversal in the aging process along with a reduction in fat and increase in muscle mass.[3]

Numerous physicians have reported similar results by augmenting HGH therapy.[4-6] Yet, the high cost of HGH injections makes it too expensive to be used by the majority of Americans. However, you can achieve the same effect at a fraction of the cost using natural substances to stimulate an increased production of HGH. In chapters 8 and 9, we will provide a guide to all the nutrients that release HGH in the body, allowing you to use safe, effective, natural substances to bring back surging HGH and IGF-1 levels, allowing you to have a sleeker, stronger, and younger body.

## PHARMACEUTICAL BOOSTERS OF HGH AND IGF-1

As we approach the millennium we enter a new era of amazing possibilities in the field of anti-aging medicine. Even the pharmaceutical industry is working aggressively on many new anti-aging pharmaceuticals and advanced hormone delivery systems.

Already many scientists are researching innovative ways to help the body release HGH and IGF-1 better than having injections of HGH which are expensive and short-lasting. As we age, HGH declines along with another hormone called Growth Hormone Releasing Hormone (GHRH) which precedes the release of HGH and IGF-1 in the body. By boosting GHRH, there is a powerful umbrella effect that causes the body to release HGH and IGF-1 levels dramatically. Emiliano Corpas,

M.D. at the John Hopkins University School of Medicine, found that GHRH injections restored HGH and IGF-1 levels in older men to that of men three decades younger.

Other researchers believe that IGF-1 therapy may be even more powerful that GHRH in increasing lean body mass, reducing fat, building muscle and bone strength.

In certain individuals who have an exhausted pituitary gland, the injection of IGF-1 may prove to bypass the weak pituitary gland, thus providing a promising way to improve glucose metabolism and regenerate nerves.

Because IGF-1 and HGH control so many anti-aging mechanisms of the body, the primary focus of LII's nutritional protocol is to enhance the natural production of these hormones. When IGF-1 levels are maintained at healthy levels, insulin levels and glucose metabolism improves, thereby decreasing the tendency of protein breakdown in the liver and gut as explained previously.

Another approach used to augment HGH activity is found in the protein-based compounds called secretagogues. Secretagogues have been clinically tested with great success. Hexuralin, a six-amino acid peptide secretagogue formula by Pharmacia Upjohn is now being tested at the University of Turin in Italy. New exciting prospects for the first oral secretagogue drug is now being researched by Merck and Company in Rahway, New Jersey. Other pharmaceutical companies are working on transdermal patches that provide the body with safe and continuous levels of HGH-releasing secretagogues.

As promising as all these new drug developments are, it may be years before these clinical trials are completed and the FDA approves these products. But you do not have to wait a decade to supplement with growth hormone releasing nutritional factors. Studies have shown that certain amino acids like glutamine, arginine and lysine increase HGH levels by 15 percent. When these amino acids are combined with precise peptide formations of biologically active proteins, IGF-1 and HGH levels increase dramatically, and in some cases, IGF-1 levels exceed the effects of having injections of HGH or IGF-1.

LII has developed a breakthrough protein powder that can be used as "meal replacement" formula for overweight individuals or as a supplement with meals. Using a proprietary method of enhancing and controlling the hydrolysis of peptide secretagogues, LII has developed a superior method of enhancing HGH and IGF-1 levels that also maintains the balance between acid and alkaline, insulin and glucagon, and preserves the integrity of the genetic blueprint. Furthermore, in addition to precise peptide formations that mimic HGH, this formula contains amino acid analogues to boost thyroid hormone production.

Genetic regulation becomes impaired with age. Every function of the cell is based on proteins. Advancing age causes protein turnover to decline throughout the cell. Balanced genetic regulation results from the LII supplement plan which strikes at the very heart of the aging process: Faulty genetic regulation. For example, when cells fail to regulate cell division, we degenerate and die. On the other hand, faulty genetic regulation causes cells to divide excessively to the point of causing cancer.

When genetic regulation is enhanced, cells become responsive to hormonal messengers and begin to upregulate their functions to optimal levels. Most importantly, this process results in vast improvements in the quality of life. Faced with a choice of living your last 30 years with aches and pains and other age-associated diseases or a vibrant healthy life, which would you choose?

The LII Anti-Aging Plan gives us the precious opportunity to improve the quality and length of our lives and those whom we love and cherish. But with this opportunity comes the personal responsibility of adhering to the day-to-day details of the LII Anti-Aging Plan.

Look at your feelings and your thoughts, and make a commitment for a longer and healthier life. Avoid turning to fads and sensational claims made by popular authors and manufacturers that have not been researched and tested for clinical effectiveness by LII. Make decisions in line with LII-tested anti-aging programs outlined in this book because these are designed to give you the maximum life span according to the latest technological advances in the field of anti-aging medicine.

Preliminary studies with LII's state-of-the-art secretagogue-based nutritional formula are impressive and it will take about a year before we know the exact details regarding actual age-reversal effects on our biomarker tests. Our best guess? We estimate that this ground-breaking formula may boost anti-aging hormone by almost 50 percent! Compared to the cost of $40 a day for synthetic HGH injections, SynchroPower™ costs a lot less and averages about $1.50 per day or 50 cents for each meal.

Scientists at LII address hormonal regulation and the interrelationships between various organs, systems and cellular networks of the body by correcting functional weaknesses caused by the aging process. By providing individuals with the foods and nutrients that improve liver function we can prevent aging and maximize our treatment protocols. Why is this so important?

Aging and age-related disorders occur long before pathology or disease can be medically diagnosed. Replacing depleted hormones while nourishing glands with natural substances restores a synchronous correlation between all bodily systems.

## DHEA AND PREG REPLACEMENT THERAPY

DHEA levels decline with aging, stress and infection. As explained previously in this chapter, PREG is a precursor to DHEA exerting actions as steroid hormone mediator in the pathway to sex hormone synthesis. The key to controlling aging is to buffer the aging-effects of stress-produced adrenal hormones. PREG and DHEA supplementation seem to control the overproduction of stress hormones. In addition, clinical success with lupus, fatigue and depression with DHEA therapy are reported in medical literature. In addition, some studies on DHEA reveal that it can reverse age-related symptoms of memory loss and cognitive function, making it a superior anti-aging hormone.[7-11]

The debate continues over which form of DHEA will yield the best and safest clinical results. Our research reveals that almost 80 percent of DHEA and PREG contain harmful solvents and other impurities. As more clinical data mounts, it is becoming more evident that synthetic or isolated forms of DHEA are not as effective as high-grade, non-toxic, yam-derived forms of DHEA and PREG. In many clinical trials, we have determined that the combined use of PREG, DHEA, and natural hormone precursors has demonstrated superior clinical results.

These extraordinary successes, documented by increased serum levels of both DHEA and PREG, are a result of using forms of PREG and DHEA that activate the biochemical pathways of PREG and DHEA formation. **Figure 13** illustrates how maintaining PREG levels results in the maximum transport and function of all steroid hormones.

In other words, the combination of DHEA and PREG reduces the amount of hormones needed to exert maximum anti-aging effects.

Immune regulatory functions also improve with this therapeutic approach, preventing the physical and mental decline associated with the aging process. When glands tire out, the use of "isolated" hormone replacement therapy results in quick short-term improvement of hormonal regulation and allows exhausted glands to rest, repair and regenerate. However, the opposite is true of long-term hormone replacement therapy—whereby glands need precursor nutrients to produce hormones and will degenerate from non-use.

Since the adrenal gland (stress-reacting and fighting gland) and pituitary gland influence the body's rate of metabolism, enhancing the body's metabolic rate helps to decrease many age-related symptoms. Indeed, thyroid function improves when precursor nutrients are administered.

## MELATONIN REPLACEMENT THERAPY

Kenichi Kitani, M.D. of the University of Tokyo stated "...since this is an endogenous hormone, the supplementation of the hormone may suppress the endogenous secretion by a feed-back mechanism. The consequence of long-term administration of melatonin, thus, needs a careful check-up in the future." Studies show that there are important reasons to question the long-term safety of taking too much melatonin.[12-15] If you take melatonin, be sure to have a physician monitor your blood and saliva levels to prevent overdosing and toxicity.

First, very little is known about the long-term effects of taking melatonin on a hormone that the latest research has found to be just as important as melatonin; epithalamin. At this point, considering the elaborate feedback loops of the pineal gland, "melatonin alone" supplementation could depress critical epithalamin levels as well as the other precious, life-extending compounds produced by the pineal gland. Another such critical compound produced by the pineal gland is TRH. This compound protects the thymus gland (major center for immunity) and improves immune system function.

Epithalamin, researched by Russian scientists, is a critical life-extending, fat-burning and immune boosting hormone. In many ways, especially with it's ability to restore fertility in test animals, epithalamin could prove to be superior to melatonin.

Due to these important studies, at this point, the only safe course for individuals concerned with life-extension would be to take pineal compounds that contain both melatonin and epithalamin along with the specific hormone precursors and nutrients to support pineal gland regulation. Until research dictates otherwise, it is only logical and reasonable to assume that long-term usage of "melatonin-alone" may disturb many vital regulatory routines of the pineal gland by depressing it's other anti-aging functions, hormones and compounds.[23,24]

Secondly, there is a critical ratio between melatonin and serotonin. Serotonin is a critical neurotransmitter responsible for a wide range of activities within the body. An excess of serotonin and a deficiency of melatonin have been linked to emotional disorders and depression. A depletion of serotonin by excessive melatonin supplementation could disturb serotonin metabolism!

Clinical studies with melatonin supplementation versus using melatonin with pineal-produced compounds, although not conclusive, seem to suggest that "melatonin alone" supplementation may upset the serotonin-melatonin ratio. There is no question of long-term safety when melatonin is combined with the hormone precursors and nutrients that strengthen pineal gland function while supplying the body with other pineal-produced anti-aging factors.

Melatonin synthesis declines with aging. Future research will have to study the levels of other vital pineal-produced hormones and compounds as the body ages. Both melatonin and epithalamin enter cells and subcellular compartments and protect intracellular molecules from oxidative damage. The ability of melatonin to enter subcellular compartments in order to effectively quench the hydroxyl radicals makes it a potent antioxidant and lifespan extender.

POINTS TO REMEMBER...

♦ Boosting HGH and IGF-1 levels while organizing and restoring control of the neuroendocrine orchestra results in superior age-reversal effects.

♦ HGH initiates the transport of proteins and nucleic acids into the body's cellular soup which helps the DNA repair itself better.

♦ HGH speeds the entry of nutrients into our cellular soup where they can be used for cell renewal and restoration.

♦ Lowering LDL and elevating HDL cholesterol enhances the production and activity of all steroid hormones.

WHAT YOU CAN DO NOW

♦ Start eating more of the age-reversing foods listed in Chapter 9.

♦ Avoid animal fats that elevate LDL cholesterol and block the production of DHEA and other vital anti-aging hormones.

♦ Remember to exercise daily to stimulate HGH production.

♦ If you're taking single hormone therapies like DHEA or melatonin, start cutting back on your doses. Have saliva tests done to determine your the correct dose for these hormones. Taking too high a dose can block the production of other very important anti-aging hormones and disturb the delicate balance of your neuroendocrine system.

♦ Concentrate on Chapter 8 to learn more about the powerful effect of secretagogues in boosting your body's natural production of HGH and IGF-1.

# CHAPTER 7

# PROSPECTS FOR THE GENETIC CONTROL OF AGING

Old age and its associated illnesses are not inevitable! Reported breakthroughs in Anti-Aging Medicine have resulted in the development of therapies that promise to overturn the tyranny of aging. These stunning medical breakthroughs promise to extend human lifespan and give individuals a life whose quality resembles that of youth in both appearance and function.

Although aging may be a part of our genetic makeup, it doesn't need to entail sickness and a slow, progressive degeneration of our bodies. Much of what we attribute to aging is a by-product of our own neglect or inability to decide what is best for our bodies in terms of how we live our lives and make our food choices.

The Human Genome Project, launched only five and a half years ago, represents a 3-billion federal effort to analyze the human genetic makeup in its ultimate molecular detail.[1] Technologies developed in response to this project have already quadrupled the rate of discovery of human disease genes. Progress is outstripping expectations as the chemical subunits of a gene are determined every hour. Throughout the next decade, this ongoing tidal wave of genetic data will help to predict how likely a person is to develop age-associated illnesses—prompting Anti-Aging physicians to prescribe appropriate life-extending therapies.

Many doctors maintain that cells and tissue invariably become weak and damaged as we age, and many disorders are hopeless, progressive and incurable. These doctors commonly state that 30 percent of people over the age of eighty die of "natural causes." However, many of these studies are not reliable as losses in physiological function due to aging cannot be measured with an autopsy. Furthermore, only 5 percent of those over eighty are autopsied.[2-6]

Many are led to believe that they should expect to lose their hearing or eyesight as they get older. Doctors blame these ailments on the aging process—but many of these disorders can be overcome. There are many civilizations in the world where people live well past 110 years of age without losing their hearing or experiencing the use of corrective eye glasses.

A whole new approach to nutrition and nutraceutical medicine, Quantum Nutrition, may finally help humans to overcome many problems related to health and longevity. Chapter 8 details the components of Quantum Nutrition and tells you how to use it to put the brakes on aging.

There you will learn about the exciting new wave of biotechnology and chemistry that enhances the body's production of youth-generating hormones. Imagine feeling decades younger and being charged with vitality as the signs of old age begin to fade away.

LII-based research in the field of Quantum Nutrition has made ground-shaking discoveries about how the body produces hormones by way of enzymes and critical nutrients—the essential components of hormone production and metabolism.

Step-by-step, information given in the coming chapters explains how to get an abundance of these hormone-producing nutrients, enzymes and natural proteins—needed to restore cells to youthful states. Understanding the molecular chemistry of aging means replacing parts of human chemistry that are missing and restoring function that is lost due to premature aging.

Understanding how the body ages and produces hormones could resolve a long-standing puzzle in biology—why and how we age. The LII Anti-Aging Plan reveals the many factors that may play a role in protecting the body's cells against the ravages of aging.

## GENETICS AND BIOMOLECULAR AGING

Because aging takes place in the microscopic cellular domain, it has attracted scientists in the fields of both molecular biology and physics. Since the 1950's genetic research has dominated thinking about the causes of aging. Changes in genes, known as mutations, and the cross-linking of proteins impede vital metabolic processes by obstructing the passage of nutrients and wastes into and out of cells. Cross-links are also known to damage nucleic acids, the very material of which our genes are composed. The genetic hypothesis of aging proposes that the consequences of genetic cross-linking are what cause genes to make mistakes in the formation of new molecular structures and proteins, producing what we know as age-related deterioration of the body.

The cross-linking of tissues, tendons, ligaments, cartilage, and skin causes our skin to become less soft and pliable and wrinkled as we age. Scientists at LII and the American Academy of Anti-Aging Medicine are even now discovering new ways to control the body's "genetic clocks" with unique nutritional and hormonal therapies. Already there is much evidence that protection of the genetic code through nutrition may be possible.

Dr. Lester Packer, of the University of California at Berkeley, has found that antioxidants, such as vitamin E, may rewire individual genetic programming and double the lifespan of cells through his controlled laboratory experiments.[7]

Contrary to the idea that often prevails, many types of illnesses are seldom caused solely by heredity. Genetic weaknesses can only predispose individuals to develop certain kinds of disorders—by making them highly vulnerable to stress from poor diet and environmental factors. Many of these environmental and dietary triggering agents that accelerate the aging process can be eliminated or decreased early in an individual's life, reducing an individual's susceptibility to the development of age-related disorders.

Genetic weaknesses may also predispose individuals to have smaller, less efficient endocrine glands, organs and circulatory systems, as well as different digestion and absorption capabilities, which can aggravate or cause many forms of what medicine calls "age-related" disorders. It should be noted that many individuals inherit long-term deficiencies and biochemical imbalances that end up causing many types of functional deficits. Put simply, instead of inheriting a disease or specific type of bodily malfunction, people inherit the deficiency that causes a certain part of their body to malfunction.

Many brilliant scientists are making amazing genetic discoveries by decoding, letter by letter, the message contained in genes. They study the basic structure of proteins, the metabolism of enzymes and activity of hormone receptors on the surface of cells. At the same time, other scientists are helping us understand more about DNA-containing chromosomes and their four telomeres or "arms" which serve as the time clocks of aging sequences.

With advancing age, the telomere shrinks and shortens in length. The progressive shrinking of the telomere eventually causes cells to stop dividing, which causes the body to age and die. Since the telomere also functions to protect the chromosome from damage and allows for the replication of chromosomes in the process of controlling gene expression, nourishing our cellular soup to keep the telomere from shrinking is an important accomplishment of the LII Anti-Aging Plan.

Recently, geneticists have made huge strides toward understanding how mutant genes can cause many common diseases. In 1995 alone, they discovered new genes that cause cataracts, prostate cancer, male infertility, Alzheimer's disease, schizophrenia and breast cancer.

Mutations in genes have multiple effects, causing repair genes to be damaged and abnormal protein sequences to be to produced. Scientists now estimate that there could be as many as 10,000 of our genes called transcription factors that code the sequence for the production of protein. These transcription factors are controlled by a communication process. Leading physicists who are studying the wave nature of atoms call the communication regulators <u>enhancers</u> that facilitate transcription and <u>silencers</u> that inhibit transcription. Like the ignition switch to your car, <u>enhancers</u> act as a conductor sparking the gene into action. <u>Silencers</u> are like the brake pedal of a car that slows down or stops transcription.

97

Cutting-edge research from Austrian and German physicists has examined the nature of atoms and the regulatory activities of the electromagnetic realm. Their discovery: when atomic waveforms are out of phase they can cause a functional decline in signal transaction. Not good! But, what throws these atoms out of phase? Deficiency states of individual cellular membrane phospholipids and proteins are the most probable causes of these phase shifts. When a defective protein binds to DNA sequences, a complex modulation of molecular events begins to occur—throwing the waveforms of many critical atoms out of phase. Since atoms make up molecules and molecular structure, it becomes obvious how this sequence of events can interfere with the proper genetic transcription of protein.

The most common source of interference comes from our modern-age electrical environment. Satellite transmissions, the rapid development of radio and television technology, computers, microwaves and X-rays all can interfere with genetic transcription—disrupting atomic forms and causing mutations in many of our genes. These interference waveforms act like molecular plugs that block critical enhancer and silencer elements—creating unwanted, inaccurate and weak transcription. When electromagnetic pollution is combined with the other functional disorders of the body, faulty genetic (enzymatic) processing of protein contributes to a vicious cycle of accelerated aging.

## THE ROLE OF PROTEIN AND DNA

Enzymes, not functioning at their full biological capacity, can make errors in their manufacturing of protein and DNA. Even an infinitesimally small error in reproducing one DNA can render it flawed and useless. Geneticists have discovered that humans possess at least six DNA repair systems. Studies have conclusively documented that the more efficient DNA-related repair network, the longer we live.

Protein can be damaged by the excessive consumption of dietary sugars that accelerate the rate of protein damage (cross-linking process). These sugar-damaged proteins become trapped in tissues and organs—causing them to age prematurely. Furthermore, the special sensors on cell membranes are made of protein and are also damaged by these sugars. Chapter 9 describes how the Anti-Aging Diet™ can be used to prevent uncontrolled blood sugars from damaging vital proteins.

From a nutritional perspective, the biochemical basis of disease and dysfunction presents no fundamental difference in many parts of the human body. Our cells need not only water, oxygen, and a suitable ambient temperature, but a precise combination of over 40 nutrients. The body's cells will ultimately get from the blood only those nutrient elements furnished by its daily intake of food.

Because of nutrient needs, enzyme patterns, biochemistry, anatomy, blood circulation, and the various types of age-related dysfunctions may vary from person to person, successful nutritional support must be derived from organic-enzymatic complexes made up of special nutrients. Ideally, each person should be evaluated as a whole and unique person with specific diet, nutrition, exercise and relaxation programs designed to meet his or her unique and individual needs.

Nutrients work together as a team and the body's cells depend upon the total spectrum of those nutrients, to protect the genetic code and activate the concise repair networks of the body. A scarcity and/or excess of only one single nutrient can reduce the efficiency of all the nutrients with which it is teamed. All nutrients are essential links in the total collection of nutrients needed by the cells of the body and must be present in sufficient amounts to function as a weapon against the ravages of aging.

## QUANTUM PHYSICS AND THE GENETIC WORLD

The field of quantum physics—examines biological processes and the aging process in the submolecular domain—the hidden world of tiny atoms. Many of these biological processes promise to answer some of the most challenging questions regarding how the body ages. The following section will give a brief overview of some of these discoveries, especially those that offer great promise in the field of enzymatic forms to be effective in stopping or slowing the progressive nature of most age-related disorders.

It is known that a healthy cell changes its function by responding to the balance of stimulatory and inhibitory signals from the neuroendocrine orchestra. Free radicals cause cells to become less responsive to these external messages, and therefore to defer vital regulatory routines. When cells become deaf to external messages, genetic mutations can lead to uncontrollable replication resulting in accelerated aging of the human organism.

Scientists believe that these malfunctioning cells are the ones that replicate uncontrollably, damaging healthy tissue and invading barriers that separate one organ from another— thereby metastasizing and establishing new colonies at distant sites.[8]

100

Research of this process over the past 20 years has identified many genes that take part in the development of cancer.[8,9] The ongoing research is confirming that cancer develops because cells suffer irreversible damage to these particular classes of genes. In addition, it is well established that over or under production of one or more proteins is found in the majority of today's illnesses. Furthermore, physicists have documented that the protein structures of the extracellular matrix amplify, transduce, and transmit minute energies that serve to control the vital regulatory routines of the body.

Mutations in genes have multiple the effects of causing repair genes to be damaged and also causing abnormal proteins to reduce the ability of cells to limit blood vessel formation. The process by which normal cells age or become cancerous is undoubtedly even more complicated at the biomolecular level where researchers have discovered several complex, multisystem issues of cellular communication or signal transduction. Insights put forth by the world's leading quantum physicists point the way to practical benefits for individuals in search of longevity.

## QUANTUM NUTRITION AND CELLULAR RESONANCE

Previously, you have discovered how the neuroendocrine orchestra functions to keep us young and healthy. In addition to the chemical communication of hormones and the electrical communication of the nervous system, the neuroendocrine orchestra also communicates electromagnetically. Just as invisible electronic signals travel through the air to a satellite dish and bring 150 television channels into your home, cells communicate via oscillations, known as biophotons.

Biophotons are the smallest particles of energy and they function deep within the genetic control centers of the body.

Molecules of DNA and cellular structures actually vibrate with subtle oscillations of energy. When these oscillations are just right they radiate very specific harmonic oscillations that help to fine-tune, stabilize, and amplify hormone transmission and reception within the body.

If all this sounds far-fetched, you would also be surprised to learn that many successful homeopathic medicines used by thousands of physicians worldwide, work on the very same energetic principles. Oscillations from homeopathic remedies excite the body's cells to perform their work more efficiently.

From a scientific perspective, there is much serious research on record to document the principle of cellular resonance. The principle of cellular resonance was documented by numerous researchers beginning in the 1970's.[10-13] In 1974, Dr. McClare stated; "There is a level of organization in biological systems—a tuned resonance between energy levels in different molecules—that enables biological systems to function rapidly and yet efficiently."[11]

In 1979, Professor Rapp in his book, An Atlas of Cellular Oscillators, cited over 450 studies that detail how "oscillations in enzyme-catylized reactions (protein synthesis) are multi-leveled series of interacting systems and subsystems that resonate harmoniously."[12]

Classical methods of molecular spectroscopy have documented that biological molecules exhibit oscillations at very specific frequencies. Nobel prize winners, Dr.

Erwin Neher and Dr. Bert Sackmann wrote "almost all physiological reactions of the cell are regulated by means of energetic impulses."

Leading Russian physicist, Dr. Lakhousky has defined life as "...the dynamic equilibrium of all cells and the harmony of multiple radiations reacting upon one another."[13]

Despite the awesome complexity of quantum physics, understanding the basic principles of cellular resonance will take you well beyond the current nutritional therapies to produce truly superior anti-aging effects. Like a fine-tuned musical instrument that produces thrilling harmonic resonances, the neuroendocrine orchestra needs both physical nourishment and energetic nourishment to resonate properly.

At LII, we define this unique combination of age-fighting nutrients and energetic resonances as Quantum Nutrition.

There is mounting evidence that these cellular resonances can and do penetrate deeply within the genetic control centers of the cells.[14-18] Specifically, this means that Quantum Nutrition protects the integrity of our cells by snuffing out the youth-stealing, free radicals that corrupt the genetic material of our cells. The staggering truth is that these incredible, energy-packed nutrients strike at the very heart of the aging process in the molecular biology of our cells. These anti-aging agents are super-charged with harmonic resonances that are imprinted or programmed into the nutritional products, allowing nutrients to penetrate the body's cells at incredible speeds and with amazing efficiency. These nutrients and their molecularly programmed resonances work in harmony to combat aging within the genetic control centers of the body, allowing individuals to live at their fullest capacity throughout their lives.

This amazing discovery, unaddressed by many of today's popular anti-aging and nutritional therapies, provides a superior defense strategy against premature aging.

The science of simple chemistry takes no account of the subtle yet necessary quantum effects needed by the body's cells or to understand the motions of molecules and the precise interactions that occur between the individual cells of the body. Aging cells become inefficient, generating large quantities of useless byproducts *(toxins and deranged proteins)*. These toxins and mutilated proteins generate dysharmonic resonances that lead to states of advanced molecular and tissue aging.

Using programmed energies to steer the right chemical reactions down a preferred pathway keeps the neuroendocrine system functioning more efficiently.

How do we know this is possible?

Researchers have documented that chemical bonds are strongly interdependent on the energy flowing between bonding sites.[19] Chemical bonds vibrate to these bursts of energy! Subsequently, cellular function and communication improves when energetic functions of the cells are enhanced with harmonic resonances.

For the first time, LII scientists are beginning to assess the issues of how particles such as electrons, atoms and molecules can behave as biophoton energies to dictate and control the anti-aging mechanisms of the body. Experiments have fully confirmed the existence of these photon-molecular reactions.[19,20]

## QUANTUM PHYSICS: FUTURE PROSPECTS FOR LONGEVITY

Research aimed at understanding and ultimately manipulating the biophoton domain that regulates protein synthesis promises to clarify some central mysteries of the individual genome and the transcription of genes.

When a protein binds to DNA sequences, biophoton frequencies regulate and modulate the molecular dynamics of our cells. Biophoton energy drives transcription and assembly of some 50 distinct proteins of the DNA. These proteins plug into receptive sockets of DNA telling it which genes can be transcribed and how quickly. Solid evidence documents that DNA is a photon storage site that controls enzymatic activity, repair, immunological functions and genetic control of both transcription and replication of DNA *(Popp, Electromagnetic Bio-Information)*.

Dr. Popp and numerous other physicists have shown that DNA-derived biophotons traveling through the cell provide what may be the fundamental mechanism of genetic control and homeostasis.[13]

The wave function, described by physicists, embodies all currently available information about the state of a biophotonic motion or dynamics. Like light bulbs, atoms emit radiant biophoton-energy that can create constructive or destructive molecular effects. In the case of destructive interference, waveforms of many biophoton emissions are out of phase — thereby causing the functional decline of the extracellular matrix and cellular membrane signaling systems. Interference waveforms produce disharmonic frequencies or dysfunctional signals that disturb biorhythms that represent the basis of all physiological functions in the body.

Interference waveforms, derived from the our modern-age electrical environment *(Robert Becker, M.D., Cross Currents, 1994)* are involved in the aging process. Since the body's detoxification mechanisms are controlled by signal transduction, toxicity of the extracellular matrix, described by Alfred Pischinger, M.D. may affect about 80% of the entire mass of body cells.[21] When the extracellular matrix is toxic and resonating with interference waveforms, faulty enzymatic processing of protein and the accumulation of amyloid beta protein in the extracellular and lymphatic system accelerate free radical-mediated damage to the body.

The implantation of interference waveforms within the cell causes irritation of the chromosomes, leading to allergic disorders or inflammatory disorders of the skin, lungs, kidneys or bowels. As implantation continues, the body implants or stores more toxins causing the cell nucleus to enlarge. Nucleus enlargement leads to the multiplication of cells *(tumor growth)* and rapid states of accelerated aging. If the implantation of these toxic waveforms is stopped early in the stages of illness, by nourishing the body with Quantum Nutrition, many toxic waveforms are discharged thus activating immunity and augmenting the healing and repair mechanisms of the cell and body.

## ELECTROMAGNETIC NEUROHORMONAL BLOCKERS

Scientists have also come to believe that melatonin can be diminished by excessive exposure to electromagnetic fields (EMFs) in the environment. EMFs are radiated by invisible energy that flow out from power lines and electrical appliances. Studies have reported that users of EMF-emitting electric blankets, have measurably lower levels of melatonin.[22,23]

But what do EMFs have to do with hormone activity? Scientists have done laboratory testing with a medical imaging device called an NMR (nuclear magnetic resonance spectroscopy) on electric blanket users and found lowered melatonin levels and abnormal magnetic resonances in some people. More compelling evidence comes from studies done by applying EMFs to guinea pigs. When these animals are exposed to EMFs, the electrical activity of the pineal gland is reduced by as much as 50 percent.[24]

These discoveries and many others have inadvertently uncovered another critical function of the pineal gland. As the pineal gland synchronizes the twenty-four-hour time period, it also triggers the body's seasonal changes and has an electromagnetic dimension of functioning!

When migrating birds are subjected to EMFs, they head North to Alaska instead of South for the winter. Homing pigeons subjected to artificial EMF's find it difficult to find their way home. Some scientists suspect that the pineal glands of whales subjected to EMFs may cause them to beach themselves in shallow lagoons.[25]

When the pineal gland and brain are cross-wired by the confusing effects of EMFs, the cellular resonance of brain cells becomes disorganized and short-circuited. Studies have documented a number of statistical links between sudden changes in the earth's magnetic field and human health problems. One such study published in Nature Magazine documented that surges in magnetic activity from solar storms are directly correlated to a higher incidence of heart attacks.[26]

## PROTECTING GENES FROM EMFS

The scientific literature is abundant with studies that link EMF's to many age-associated diseases. If research is showing that EMFs are harmful to the pineal gland and body, what can we do to fortify the body and protect it from the aging effects of harmful EMFs?

While some scientists claim we should find ways to avoid EMFs altogether, others claim these man-made electric fields are harmless. Those who claim EMFs are harmless have failed to properly analyze there effects on the pineal gland and the electrical dimension of the body. Avoidance of all EMFs may be impossible in today's world. However, the following precautionary steps may prove beneficial:

1   Keeping a distance from all electronic appliances in your home is helpful as EMFs decrease at distances of one to two feet.

2   Shield computer monitors with filters that reduce glare and the electrical fields of computer monitors.

3   Make sure your sleeping environment is safe. Keep any electronic devices (alarm clocks, telephone answering systems, radios and clocks) at least three feet from your bed. Avoid electric blankets and heating your water bed while you are sleeping.

4   Use battery-operated or rechargeable appliances when possible.

Until more research defines the safe limits of EMF exposure, finding ways to strengthen the body's electromagnetic connections with the pineal gland is critically important. One way to accomplish this is by applying the scientific principle of cellular resonance.

We know that interference waveforms act as molecular plugs that block genetic functions, thereby creating unwanted or weak transcription. Because interference of molecular pathways blocks important regulatory routines, the cancellation of these interference waveforms with Quantum Nutrition is very important. This is because every organ uses biophotonic waveforms to signal and harmonize the regulatory routines of the body.

Biophysical signals and steering mechanisms of the human regulatory system occur faster than the speed of light in the electromagnetic domain, providing a highly efficient means of manipulating the biomolecular domain of the body. When interference waveforms are stored in the body, namely in the extra- and intra-cellular areas, they adversely affect the DNA of the cell nuclei. The use of harmonic oscillations needed to help the internal organs and tissues regain their full efficiency and ability to function at the biomolecular level dramatically improves hormone transmission, activity, and reception.

In Germany, biophotonic light pulses (*a collection of biophotons with different energies*) represent another method of controlling the outcomes of chemical reactions. It has been demonstrated that a wide range of pulsed energies can induce motion (*vibration or rotation*) in a molecule.

Dynamic molecular changes result from the pulsed activity of the frequencies. According to many researchers, a complicated mixture of pulsed frequencies is necessary to control molecular dynamics optimally. According to Helmut Breithaupt, M.D., "the optimal interplay between multiple control circuits is, in effect, an inquiry into communication between various functional processes within the organism." Dr. Breithaupt documents that regulatory oscillations are superimposed in a three-tiered hierarchy:

1   Frequency Modulation which is employed to transfer information;

2   Phase Modulation which is involved in data processing;

3   Amplitude Modulation needed to dampen oscillations found in reactive processes of the body.

The coordination of all these oscillations takes place when the vital processes can distinguish between frequency and phase modulation. Since functional stress leads to continuous frequency modulation in the information rhythmics of the nervous, cardiac and respiratory systems, amplitude modulation plays a vital role in counteracting these stress reactions—allowing efficient adaptation to take place.

Understanding, and ultimately manipulating the regulation of protein synthesis by complex waveforms of multiple-pulsed biophotons may soon provide valuable information regarding clinical approaches for the aging dilemma and modern day illnesses.

As satisfying as the clinical results of biophoton applications are, they do not fully explain how molecular signals are conveyed and modulate transcription. Such clinical approaches are remote today, but it is exciting to consider how applications of Quantum Nutrition might eventually delay or forestall the aging process.

Therapies of the future will benefit in one way or another from the research of quantum physicists and molecular biologists as they design effective clinical protocols to conquer aging and degenerative disease.

What can the field of quantum physics tell us about the aging immune system? Future directions may include specific biophoton therapies that activate disease-fighting cells of the immune system and regenerate glands or organs that are functionally weak. At present, many leading physicists are very close to finding ways to modulate any immune function with the use of frequencies or biophoton light therapies.

The healthy immune system works in concert with a vast network of bioregulatory systems and electromagnetic circuits. These systems of biomolecular signal transduction transfer signals from protein to protein, thereby leading to a cascade of molecular reactions that lead to a change in cell behavior. These molecular states of regulatory behavior are necessary to keep the body functioning the way it was designed to function in normal or natural states of physiology. Clearly, approaches that enhance energy and increase biocommunication between the many systems of the body, will have the most success in the field of anti-aging medicine.

Quantum (*electromagnetic*) interference of molecular pathways results from the storage of toxins and the impregnation of mutilated proteins structures and trans fatty acid in the lymphatics and extracellular matrix. For a molecule to undergo the dynamics of any signal transduction process, a superposition or a sum of wave functions representing stationary states of different energies must interact favorably with it. This harmonic interaction is required to control molecular dynamics and the bioregulatory cycles of immunity optimally.

Since the specific responses a cell makes depend on the precise combination of signals affecting it from without as well as the mix of its receptors, improving bioregulation via Quantum Nutrition will provide necessary stimulus for optimal detoxification and energy enhancement.

**KEY POINTS TO REMEMBER...**

♦ The field of quantum physics provides us with new concepts in the understanding of physiological patterns involved in the aging process, a way to understand aging in the submolecular and hidden world of atoms.

♦ The concept of cellular resonance provides LII with a revolutionary way to penetrate nutrients deep into the genetic control centers of the body, allowing us to combat aging at the genetic level.

♦ As we approach the 21st century, quantum physics will continue to open up unprecedented possibilities for understanding molecular and electromagnetic processes as they relate to the advanced molecular and tissue aging.

♦ Quantum Nutrition can augment gene transcription and cellular communication (signal transduction), allowing the cell to defend its metabolic pathways from free radical attacks.

♦ Enhancing DNA synthesis through proper dietary measures, Quantum Nutritional supplementation, and avoiding toxins in our environment speeds up cellular repair mechanisms at the genetic level.

♦ Maintaining healthy, anti-aging resonance's is also enhanced when we protect our genes from EMFs.

♦ The LII Biomarker Matrix Protocol assesses biological aging on five levels: the physiological level, the cellular level, the molecular level, the chromosomal level, and the electromagnetic level.

## WHAT YOU CAN DO NOW

♦ Shield your computer monitor with a protective filter.

♦ Keep a distance of two feet from all electric appliances in your home.

♦ Avoid using a microwave to cook your foods.

♦ Avoid electric blankets and heating your water bed while sleeping.

♦ Concentrate on the information presented in Chapter 8 where you will discover the full details of Quantum Nutrition.

♦ Avoid processed, chemical-laden, and refined foods that disturb the body's natural and harmonic resonances at the cellular and genetic levels.

♦ Consult with Appendix A for a list of toxins that accelerate aging by disturbing cellular resonance and blocking many genetic and enzymatic functions.

114

# CHAPTER 8

# THE LII QUANTUM NUTRITION PLAN

Quantum Nutrition is designed to create high efficiency in all of the physiological systems of the body. By upregulating the function of aging organ systems, we increase the activity of anti-aging mechanisms and move physiological systems closer to their optimal performance. In today's toxic world, boosting reserve energies or building an extra margin of physiological capacity by fine-tuning the neuroendocrine orchestra and allowing nourishment to penetrate our individual microscopic genetic world are primary goals of the LII Anti-Aging Plan.

Quantum Nutrition, first described and researched by these authors of this book over a decade ago, can realistically contribute to health status and the quality of life beyond simply providing needed physical nutrients.[1-6] In it, the answers to many questions about human longevity as well as the physiological processes that regulate genetic transcription and the duration of life are to be found. Quantum Nutrition addresses these processes on the physiological, cellular, chromosomal, molecular, genetic, and electromagnetic levels.

As outlined previously, Quantum Nutrition offers a plausible program for obtaining optimal longevity. By improving the molecular and nutrient status of our cellular soup, we enhance the function of cell membrane receptors and activate all levels of hormone activity (**Figure 16**). After over a decade of clinical trials, it is clearly evident

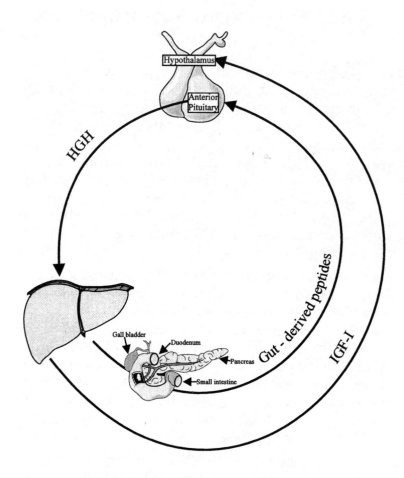

**Figure 16**. The feedback loop between liver-produced IGF-I and the hypothalamus in the brain to direct the pituitary to make more HGH. HGH produced from gut-dervied peptides stimulates the liver to produce IGF-I.

that the quality of life improves dramatically with this form of advanced nutritional support.

Significant amounts of energy are needed to maintain the accuracy of molecular processes such as the replication and repair of DNA as well as the synthesis and turnover of proteins. These well documented facts make it worthwhile for an individual in search of maximized longevity to seek out higher levels of nutritional maintenance, designed to preserve vital functions well beyond normal levels. An extra reserve of nutritional factors leaves individuals with the high reserves of energy needed to deal with today's higher stress levels and ever increasing environmental pollution.

The emerging picture of the genetic mechanism of longevity suggests that nutritional factors regulate the efficiency of anti-aging systems. Aging is the result of the progressive depletion of vital anti-aging nutrients which causes a deterioration of genetic and cellular maintenance processes. Remember that, when energy becomes scarce, the body resorts to cannibalistic functions by robbing the protein or minerals it needs from itself. To make matters worse, these low energy states invite free radical renegades to attack the basic units of life: cells.

## SYNCHRONIZING THE NEUROENDOCRINE ORCHESTRA

The evidence being presented in this book builds a very strong case for Quantum Nutrition and the LII Anti-Aging Diet as the primary means of synchronizing and fine-tuning neuroendocrine orchestrations, building the body's antioxidant defenses, and protecting the genetic blueprint.

A problem of fundamental importance in understanding cellular senescence is grasping an adequate knowledge of the mechanisms by which cells communicate with one another via harmonic resonances. Considering quality of life issues from the perspective of the Quantum Nutrition, we need to define health and the quality of life beyond the physical perspective. This broader perspective of thinking addresses the full complexity of the aging process as it is being defined by leading biomolecular scientists and physicists.

In regard to the tuning of the body's neuroendocrine orchestra, regulation of endocrine, paracrine, autocrine, and intracrine activity is achieved by establishing tight controls and maintaining the status of hormone receptors. Careful study and ongoing scientific research have led LII to develop precise Quantum Nutritional formulas that represent a major breakthrough beyond simple multivitamins. These formulas are designed to support anti-aging defenses on four levels:

1    Protein Nutrition: benefits function of bioactive peptides and amino acid analogue hormones
2    Lipid And Fatty Acid Nutrition: enhances steroid hormone pathways
3    Antioxidant Nutrition
4    Quantum Nutrition

## PROTEIN NUTRITION: BIOACTIVE PEPTIDES AND AMINO ACIDS

Over the last few decades, the emphasis in the nutritional field has been primarily in viewing protein nutrition in the form of amino acids. For a long time nutritional scientists believed that only amino acids entered the body's circulation through the gut. Current evidence indicates that bioactive peptides, known as secretagogues, also possess unique and powerful anti-aging actions within the organism.[7-22] Secretagogues can alter cellular metabolism by acting as hormones or neurotransmitters. **Figure 17** illustrates how gut-derived peptides are part of a feedback loop that stimulates the pituitary gland to produce HGH. In turn, when HGH reaches the liver, IGF-1 is also produced from these peptides. Peptides are hydrolyzed protein fragments that cross the small intestine and reach cells via systemic circulation.

Bioactive peptides dictate a variety of metabolic responses in the neuroendocrine orchestra. Studies have reported that these very same peptides are superior to free form amino acids and can improve immune function, lower blood pressure, and shorten recovery time after an illness. This form of protein can improve gut function and absorption. Thousands of patients with gut permeability problems and malabsorption have benefited from the use of bioactive peptides.[23-28]

As you may recall from earlier study, many hormones HGH, IGF1, insulin, and glucagon are peptides. These peptides possess high levels of biological activity. Shorter peptides have different physiological functions than longer peptides. For example, Thyroid Stimulating Hormone (TSH) produced by the pituitary gland uses longer peptides, while the thyroid gland produces hormones from amino acid analogues.

According to up-to-date research, the longer peptides are also involved in hormonal transmission. The pituitary gland uses peptide hormones (TSH, FSH, ACTH, HGH) to keep the neuroendocrine orchestra synchronized.

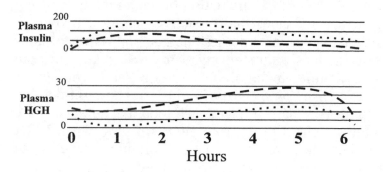

**Figure 17.** Suboptimal(— —) versus optimal(· · ·) HGH concentrations as a function of insulin levels over a 6 hour time period.

Likewise, hormonal transmission is governed by both frequency and amplitude modulation. In other words, the frequency and concentration of peptide-generated pulses determines the quantity and quality of hormonal transmission.

During prolonged periods of stress, gut circulation decreases; causing deficiencies of both peptides and amino acids. If these protein fragments are not supplemented daily, we run the risk of impairing protein synthesis and blocking many healing routines of the body.

Although many nutritional formulas contain peptides and amino acids, there are significant differences in the quantity and quality of peptides in these various formulas. The sequences of peptides need to be carefully controlled by the degree and type of hydrolysis. LII uses a proprietary method of utilizing specific enzymes to cleave protein in order to produce neuroendocrine patterns of peptides (secretagogues) and amino acid analogue activity (SynchroPower™).

120

Secretagogues and amino acids keep hormones balanced and work in conjunction with the biochemistry of the body to provide the necessary precursors to the body's cellular soup—to promote the maximum genetic blueprint preservation effects.

## LIPID AND FATTY ACID NUTRITION

Just as we need good quality proteins in the form of bioactive peptides, we also need high quality fats. There is a substantial and growing body of evidence indicating that many age-related disorders are caused by deficits in fatty acid metabolism.[28-32] Modern processing methods of fats and oils have created powerful and toxic forms of age-promoting rancid and trans fatty acids that cause the body to become deficient in the Omega-3 and Omega-6 fatty acids as well as prostaglandins, also known as ecosanoid hormones. You will learn more about food sources of fatty acids in the upcoming chapter.

Our hormones and the membranes of our cells use fats to manufacture and transport hormones. A deficiency of Omega-6 fatty acids, derived from cold water salmon, has been implicated as a main cause of inflammatory and degenerative disorders as well as other modern maladies.

Ecosanoid hormones are part of the paracrine and autocrine divisions of the neuroendocrine orchestra. Remember, paracrine and autocrine hormonal communication occurs faster than endocrine activities. These fast-acting hormones have powerful anti-aging effects. Without a sufficient supply of anti-inflammatory ecosanoid hormones, the neuroendocrine orchestra fails to function on all four levels: the endocrine, paracrine, autocrine, and intracrine.

Just like the tightrope walker is able to maintain balance by continuous action from side to side, there are two opposing forces of ecosanoid activity: age-promoting ecosanoids and age-reversing ecosanoids. Striving for a healthy balance between free radicals and antioxidants, and both kinds of ecosanoids is necessary to gain the maximum anti-aging effects.

Our studies have shown that individuals whose biological age exceeds their chronological age have excesses of age-promoting ecosanoids caused by both stress and the dietary excesses of saturated and trans fats as well as deficiencies of unsaturated Omega-6 fatty acids. In addition, the premature aging of their digestive system made it impossible for them to emulsify and digest the "good" fats and converting them into age-reversing ecosanoids. After decades of clinical trials, LII has developed a new fatty acid delivery system for supplementation that dramatically increases the body's levels of age-reversing ecosanoids (EndoSync™).

## Antioxidant Nutrition

We know that renegade free radicals wage a war against the body's cells causing tissues and organs to age rapidly. Antioxidants combat those free radicals, keeping them from attacking healthy cells, DNA, and the genetic material within the cell's nucleus. The quality of our "redox reaction" refers to this process by which free radicals are neutralized (oxidative stress). In this battlefield of the ongoing war against free radicals, we need to supplement daily with effective redox nutrients that counterattack the age-promoting free radicals thus protecting us from molecular injury.[36-40]

- To prevent free radical chain reactions, our first priority must be to upregulate redox functions and support the body's molecular defense pathways. According to our research, the following antioxidants, when used together, provide optimal redox functions in the body:

- Vitamin E - unesterified, free from soy oil, wheat germ oil, or any oil dilutant which can turn rancid and reduce redox functions;

- COQ10 is a powerful antioxidant that protects lipid-transporting hormones and fat molecules from being oxidized. COQ-10 also protects cell membranes while sparking the cell's energy factories (mitochondria) into accelerated action;

- Reduced Glutathione - a powerful antioxidant that protects cell membranes and reduces oxidative stress in the liver;

- N-Acetyl Cysteine - a precursor to glutathione;

- Pine Bark Extract - a superior antioxidant;

- Lipoic acid - Protects cell membranes and DNA from heavy metals;

- Vitamin B2 helps the body get rid of free-radical toxins like benzene;

- Zinc- activator of many antioxidant enzymes and protein synthesis;

- Antioxidant enzymes are powerful, fast-acting antioxidants that work at the molecular level.

When the above antioxidants are combined with phytochemicals found in age-reversing foods, the redox functions at a high level of anti-aging activity.

One final point on antioxidants—there is powerful synergy between all of the LII formulations. Hundreds of reactions that give rise to an optimal redox potential are governed by enzymes. When enzymes are lacking or out of sync with other nutrients, redox function is diminished. The multiple interactions between each nutrient complex creates optimal protection for your body. Each link in your body's nutritional chain of events must be strengthened, balanced and synchronized for you to preserve your genetic blueprint.

## QUANTUM NUTRITION

Before you can appreciate the value of Quantum Nutrition, it is important to view the body as an electrical system. The body's electrical wires are the invisible meridians and nerve connections that give life and function to all body organs and systems. In simple terms, it has electrical functions just like the wiring of a house.

Before an electrician even attempts to put power through an electrical circuit, he ascertains that the electrical wiring has the correct amount of resistance and insulation. Insufficient resistance or insulation can cause a short circuit or blockage of electrical energy. As we explained in the previous chapter, the human cell also may become short-circuited due to environmental factors that slow down or block many enzymes and cellular functions.

By energizing our cells with healthy resonances, we enhance those cells' ability to utilize all of the anti-aging nutrients. These resonances have the amazing ability to penetrate deep within the molecules of living cells to reach the sub-microscopic anti-aging mechanisms of the genetic world. Pure harmonic resonances are necessary to propel nutrients down deeply into the cell so they can quickly energize the cells' functions. Why is this process important? As the body grows older, it loses its ability to utilize nutrients at the cellular level. Thus, in order to stave off the undesirable effects of aging, we need easy-to-assimilate and energized forms of Quantum Nutrition.

A very effective system for enhancing the bioavailability of nutrients—the total amount that reach the cells—Quantum Nutrition accelerates enzyme functions and other cellular repair and regenerative functions in order to fight premature aging. The bottom line for any nutritional formula is how much of the nutrients are actually delivered through the blood and into the cells and genes. Assimilation of these nutrients into the molecular and genetic environment is the primary goal of anti-aging therapies.

### KEY POINTS TO REMEMBER...

♦ LII's approach to nutritional supplementation is designed to excite and unblock neuroendocrine activity and enhance genetic pathways that are deficient due to accelerated molecular and tissue aging.

♦ LII's unique formulas work with pinpoint accuracy to nourish subcellular components and direct the body to initiate the healing process.

♦ The coupling of harmonic resonances with easy-to-assimilate forms of nutrition, clears blocked biochemical pathways while correcting all shortages and neuroendocrine irregularities.

♦ The activation of many dormant regenerative functions—through the synergistic harmony of all these formulas—allows the body to effectively address the underlying causes of premature aging.

## WHAT YOU CAN DO NOW

♦ See Appendix D for Sources of Quantum Nutritional products that will preserve your genetic blueprint.

♦ Use SynchroPower™ as a meal replacement to lose weight or take it with and in between meals to maintain superior levels of HGH and IGF-1 while keeping your insulin/glucagon ratio balanced.

♦ Take EndoSync™ with each meal to keep your fast-acting ecosanoid hormones at anti-aging levels.

♦ Take Synchrox™ with each meal to provide optimal antioxidant defenses against harmful free radicals.

♦ Take PREGURSEX™ to maintain youthful levels of both PREG and DHEA.

# CHAPTER 9

# THE LII ANTI-AGING DIET PLAN

Throughout the pages of this book we have emphasized the importance of being "balanced." The LII Anti-Aging Diet Plan provides you with a "well-balanced diet plan" that will actually stabilize and balance your neuroendocrine orchestra and enhance genetic control mechanisms of your body.

With a basic understanding of the dietary factors that govern hormonal and genetic interrelationships, you can work with, rather than against your body's anti-aging defenses. By making informed choices, you will maintain a continued high-level state of wellness that synchronizes your total body.

Natural biochemical pathways that lead to the production of anti-aging hormones maintain their balance under tight control much like a tightrope walker. The internal and external stresses from our food choices or environmental stressors work like a team to knock us out of balance, and disturb our neuroendocrine orchestrations. The result: balance is under loose control, like a pendulum's wide swing. When we become aware of the wide pendulum swing effect of our diets on our bodily systems, we will understand better how to maintain proper balance continuously.

Maximum lifespan or longevity is directly related to our body's ability to maintain its balance on the following levels:

1     The Genetic Level, where quantum nutrition and our food choices nourish and protect our genetic blueprint while keeping pH control mechanisms under tight control.

2     The Cellular Soup Level, where age-promoting free radicals are kept under tight control by our food and supplement choices. Here the goal is to provide easy-to-assimilate nourishment to our body's cellular soup.

3     The Neuroendocrine Level, where hormonal balance is maintained under tight control by powerful regulatory hormones (HGH and IGF-1) which along with diet helps to balance insulin-glucagon levels.

## BEYOND THE ZONE: THE LII ANTI-AGING DIET

The LII Anti-Aging Diet, unlike the popular ZONE diet plan, focuses on maintaining equilibrium on many levels simultaneously. Focusing only on the insulin/glucagon ratio, can cause us to lose sight of the full complexity of the aging process. It is a common misconception that we get an anti-aging effect from dietary plans that only attempt to control the insulin/glucagon ratio.

When we eat a candy bar or drink several cups of coffee and feel a spaciness or lightheadedness, it is because we have upset the natural balance of our hormones, chemistry right down to the genetic level of functioning. Although many hormones react to our food choices, the most important ones effected are HGH and IGF-1. Remember, insulin and glucagon are kept under tight control by these hormones.

The Standard American Diet (we call it SAD) elevates insulin and disturbs the body's natural balance of blood sugar, pH, and hormones. Avoiding the "yo-yo" effect of eating too many refined or simple carbohydrates, simple sugars, and stimulatory substances like caffeine a major element of this type of diet. Every time dietary choices elevate insulin, they lower critical blood sugar levels. In time, the body responds to these drops in blood sugar as a stress reaction. The adrenal glands start to produce excessive amounts of adrenaline, cortisol and cortisone. These hormones then proceed to throw the entire neuroendocrine orchestra way out of tune and the body enters a vicious cycle, called the "Alarm Reaction."

In normal and natural physiology, the alarm reaction is provoked when our bodies are preparing for the threat of bodily harm or severe stress. If a bear attacks us, the alarm reaction kicks in and adrenaline gives us a quick blast of energy by changing our neuroendocrine function to a "fight or flight" mode of action.

Unfortunately, modern-day life has us constantly in the alarm reaction stage of physiology for prolonged periods of time. This dangerous cycle promotes rapid acidification of our cellular soup, causing premature molecular and tissue aging.

If you are aggressive, time-urgent, addictive, anxious, paranoid, and have a tendency to get violent or angry more than you would like, you are most likely stuck in this vicious cycle. If you are tired when you wake up in the morning and need a cup of coffee just to function, you are experiencing life in this dangerous cycle.

There is good news however: you can subdue the "alarm reaction" of your physiology and seize control of the aberrant hormonal responses that accelerate aging.

You need not be a slave to food cravings and addictions. The LII Anti-Aging Plan is not about counting calories, fasting or drastic starvation-like food reductions. You can eat large quantities of many wonderful foods and never worry about feeling hungry after a meal.

Despite numerous dietary myths that abound regarding the proper ratio of proteins, carbohydrates, and fats, there are many different types of proteins and carbohydrates. Each has its own unique positive or negative effect on the body's equilibrium. When we analyze carbohydrates, it becomes apparent that some carbohydrates have an average of 35 percent protein and about 5 percent fat—the precise ratio needed by the body to manufacture hormones and keep neuroendocrine function in excellent working order.

Although these observations contradicted conventional diet theory, after over a decade of clinical trials we learned this vital lesson: The best way to boost the anti-aging activities of the neuroendocrine system is to eat liberally from food groups that have this perfect balance.

Mother Nature has given us this perfect balance in many foods!

In these and many other clinical experiments, patients who followed the conventional diet failed to improve, remained overweight, and continued to suffer from stress-related and age-related symptoms.

The consumption of too much animal protein and its natural saturated fat content proved to be the worst enemy of all to the neuroendocrine orchestra.[1-5] Yet, the ZONE diets and many other popular hypoglycemic-type diet advocate eating more animal protein making individuals even more acidic. For the majority of patients exhibiting signs of accelerated aging, these food groups elevated LDL cholesterol to dangerously high levels, diminishing liver-based receptors that, as we have seen, pull cholesterol out of the blood.

Where does that extra cholesterol go?

It gets deposited in the lining of blood vessels, narrowing the passageways within them and reducing the flow of vital anti-aging nutrients to the body's cells.

Despite the high protein intake of their diets, these individuals were deficient in peptides and amino acids, anti-inflammatory ecosanoid hormones, and were far too acidic.

**Figure 18** illustrates how the LII Anti-Aging Diet works to maintain the optimal concentrations of HGH and insulin in the blood.[6-11] Individuals who consume high amounts of simple sugars and carbohydrates combined with too much animal protein have lower levels of HGH and higher levels of insulin. As we have already discussed in detail, HGH has a powerful stabilizing effect on insulin, causing insulin to let glucose, proteins, and fatty acids flow into our cellular soup instead of the body's cells.

## YOUR ANTI-AGING DIET

The primary goals of the LII Anti-Aging Diet Plan are to maintain the optimal balance at the genetic, cellular, and neuroendocrine levels. Although this may seem like a complex task, we have simplified this program so much that you can easily accomplish all three goals with one diet plan.

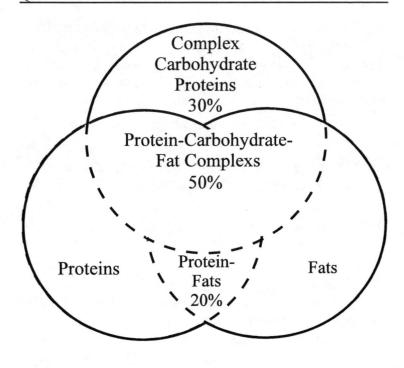

**Figure 18.** The LII Anti-Aging Diet Plan.

Plant-based protein foods or the CARBOHYDRATE - PROTEIN - FAT food groups provide us with an abundance of antioxidants and alkaline-producing and easy-to-digest proteins that maintain a healthy insulin/ glucagon ratio. The protein levels of these foods arrest the "alarm reaction" and maintain a healthy pH (acid/ alkaline balance), while stimulating the production of

HGH and IGF-1. Table 2 lists the foods that adequately accomplish this task:

## TABLE 2 - CARBOHYDRATE-PROTEIN-FAT FOOD GROUPS

| | |
|---|---|
| spinach | watercress |
| broccoli | dark green lettuce |
| kale | Brussels sprouts |
| turnip greens | mung bean sprouts |
| cauliflower | mushrooms |
| Chinese cabbage | parsley |
| zucchini | green beans |
| cucumbers | green peppers |
| artichokes | cabbage |
| celery | eggplant |
| tomatoes | onions |
| beets | bean sprouts |
| apples | grapefruits |
| grapes | dandelion greens |

By eating one or more of these foods with one or two meals daily, we maintain superior neuroendocrine and metabolic balance on many levels of functioning. This means HGH and IGF-1 levels will go up, insulin goes down, glucagon goes up, and pH is maintained at anti-aging levels in our cellular soup.

But, there are yet two more food groups that we need in order to maintain a healthy HDL and LDL cholesterol level. In review, when LDL is too high and HGH is too low, we fail to transport and manufacture steroid hormones effectively. When this happens, DHEA, testosterone, estrogen and many other hormones become deficient.

## MAINTAINING HDL AND LDL
## CHOLESTEROL AT ANTI-AGING LEVELS

Cholesterol is synthesized in the liver and by each cell of the body. According to John McDougall, M.D., our bodies produce between 500 and 1,000 milligrams of cholesterol each day. Despite the fact that our bodies create an ample supply of cholesterol, the average American consumes between 500 and 1,000 milligrams of cholesterol daily that is derived from saturated fats (meat, poultry, fish, dairy, and eggs).

It is well established that an excess of dietary cholesterol raises LDL cholesterol and contributes to the many age-related disorders that afflict Americans.[12-15] In contrast, plant-based proteins, contain no cholesterol. Instead they contain polyunsaturated and monosaturated fats. Polyunsaturated fats are found in high concentrations in the vegetables we listed for maintaining pH balance and the insulin/glucagon ratio (Table 2). Monosaturated fats come from unrefined and cold-pressed olive oil, and avocados, peanuts, and cashews.

Considering the fact that we can get all the fatty acids we need from the vegetables (Table 2), the only oil we want to consume is extra-virgin olive oil that is not bleached or otherwise subjected to any de-naturing process. Here is how to lower your risk of getting heart disease and other age-related disorders:

1    Cut back, gradually if necessary, on your intake of all animal products. Reduce and maintain your saturated fat intake to 10 percent of your overall diet.

2    Increase your intake of foods listed in Table 2.

3    Decrease your intake of simple carbohydrates and sugars, replacing them with CARBOHYDRATE-PROTEIN-FAT FOODS listed in Table 3.

4    Get most of your fats and oils in FAT-PROTEIN FOODS listed in Table 4.

5    Avoid all processed, refined, and hydrogenated oils and margarine's.

### TABLE 3. CARBOHYDRATE -PROTEIN FOODS

| | |
|---|---|
| Millet | Steel-cut oats |
| Cracked rye berries | Whole rye flakes |
| Cracked wheat berries | Wheat germ |
| Whole grain rye bread | Sprouted Grain Bread |
| Yams | Sweet potatoes |
| Lentils | Pumpkins |
| Split peas | Garbanzo beans |
| Great Northern Beans | All Legumes |

### TABLE 4. FAT-PROTEIN FOODS

| | |
|---|---|
| Pumpkin seeds | Sunflower seeds |
| Almonds | Soybeans |
| Cashews | Macadamia nuts |
| Olives | Avocados |
| Tuna | Salmon |
| Mackerel | Haddock |
| Codfish | Trout |
| Lean Meats | Soybean curd (tofu) |

**Figure 18** illustrates the percentage of each food group that you should consume to maintain maximum anti-aging effects. It's okay to eat fish, chicken, and turkey if you consume adequate amounts of the all the food groups listed above. But remember that fish, chicken,

and turkey contain saturated fats that will interfere with the transport and utilization of anti-aging hormones like PREG and DHEA. So eat small amounts of these foods in relationship to the other food groups. Always remember that the food choices listed in Table's 2-4 are age-reversing foods that can counteract the dietary mistakes you may make from time to time.

## FINE-TUNING YOUR METABOLIC BALANCE

If you are overweight and your biomarker test indicates moderate to advanced states of premature aging, you need additional help. Every time you eat take three tablespoons of SynchroPower™. You can sprinkle it on your foods, put it in oatmeal or other cooked grains, or make a delicious protein shake with your favorite fresh juice. Do this at every meal and in between meals and you will be losing stored body fat—all without food cravings and hunger.

Those with biomarker scores in the range between 30-70 can take 1 tablespoon with meals to maximize the anti-aging effects of the diet and provide their bodies with secretagogue-type peptides for boosting HGH and IGF-1 levels.

Please remember that this diet plan offers you a great deal of freedom. There are no calories to count and no food blocks of protein, fat, or carbohydrates to juggle together. You should feel free to combine any items on Table's 2-4. Just be sure to follow the basic guidelines for the relative amounts of food to consume in each group.

## SIMPLIFIED ANTI-AGING MEAL PLAN

When we developed the Anti-Aging Diet, we realized that people needed practical suggestions on what proportions of each food group to consume. The suggested menus offer vegetarian options as well as ones that contain sources of animal protein. Remember, that too much animal protein makes you acidic and elevates (the bad kind) LDL cholesterol. However, most people find they have the most energy when they avoid animal protein altogether.

By preparing in advance, you will be able to whip up tasty, healthful meals. You will need to have all the ingredients on hand to prepare these healthful recipes. It is always wise to eat one or two fresh salads daily with your lunch or dinner choices. By preparing a large bowl of salad greens on the weekend and storing these greens in a large plastic bag, you will be able to make instant salads. In addition, keep in mind that many of your dinner choices make excellent lunches the next day. In fact, you may want to cook double portions just for that purpose.

**BREAKFAST CHOICES:**

♦ A large bowl of slow-cooked steel-cut oats with 2 tablespoons of organic raisins. Use cinnamon, a dash of nutmeg and 1 tablespoon of olive oil on top.

♦ A large bowl of slow-cooked cracked rye berries. Top with raw sunflower seeds or slivered almonds.

♦ Scrambled Tofu with diced peppers, onions, turmeric, and chopped spinach. Use olive oil to sauté mixture.

♦ Raw sunflower seeds (1/2 cup) combined with 1 apple and ½ cup of water in a blender. Top with grated almonds.

## LUNCH CHOICES:

♦ A large spinach salad with 3 tablespoons of olive oil and ½ cup of raw sunflower seeds.

♦ Lentil soup (2 cups) made with lentils, vegetables and olive oil served over 1 cup of cooked cracked rye berries.

♦ Tuna on sprouted grain bread with tomato and lettuce.

♦ Grilled tofu on Rudolph's rye bread with sliced tomato and sprouts.

## DINNER CHOICES:

♦ Grilled Salmon (3 ounces) served with 3-5 cups of any combination of vegetables in Table 2.

♦ High protein (Rummo) pasta, (2 cups) primavera with your choice of any vegetable combinations from Table 2. Use olive oil to sauté vegetables. Top with romano pecorino grated cheese.

♦ Vegetables (3-4 cups) stir-fried with grilled chicken (1/2 cup). Add olive oil, herbs, and garlic to taste.

♦ String beans (3 cups) with tomato sauce served over white basmati rice. Top with romano pecorino grated cheese.

If you eat out frequently, most restaurants are happy to follow special requests. For lunch, stick to vegetable choices and salads. For dinner, choose 3-4 ounces of broiled or grilled seafood and start your meal with a large salad dressed deliciously in olive oil and vinegar. Be sure to skip the bread, butter, potatoes, and rice. Most restaurants will be happy to replace these items with cooked spinach, broccoli or other vegetables. When looking at the restaurant menu, here are some key words to look out for and avoid:

♦ creamed

♦ scalloped

♦ hollandaise

♦ deep-fried

♦ scalloped

♦ tempura

♦ fried

Remember, there is no restriction on the amount of foods you can consume from Table 2. No matter how much of these foods you eat, you will not gain weight or disturb the equilibrium of your body. Here is the most important thing to remember: Restrict your intake of foods from the Fat-Protein Table, keeping them to about 10-20 percent of each meal.

Unlike the ZONE diet, you will not have to calculate the number of blocks to eat of different foods. In fact, you carry your own high tech calculator with you at all times: the palm of your hand. Visualize consuming about four handfuls of vegetables relative to one handful of fish or lean meat; or perhaps four handfuls of vegetables relative to one handful of raw sunflower seeds or slow-cooked oatmeal and you will stay right on target!

Always remember that your intake of foods from Table 2 should be half or more of each meal. To make it easier, use the following template:

| 50% Protein-Carbohydrate-Fat | 30% Carbohydrate-Protein | 10-20% Protein-Fat |
|---|---|---|
| 1. Salad | Rye Bread | Sunflower Seeds, Olive oil |
| 2. Stir-fried Vegetables | Cracked Rye berries | Tofu and Olive oil. |
| 3. Grilled eggplant with tomato | Pasta (egg-free) | Olive oil, grated cheese |
| 4. Green beans & tomato sauce | Wheat berries | Slivered raw almonds |
| 5. Artichoke hearts, sun-dried tomatoes | Pasta with basil | Olive oil |
| 6. Spinach Salad | Rye bread | Grilled Fish or chicken |
| 7. Grapefruit | Steel-cut oatmeal | Sesame or sunflower seeds |
| 8. Lentil-Vegetable soup | Swedish rye crackers | Tofu |

And, what about snacks? You will not really need to snack if your taking your protein powder with and in-between each meal. Remember, your body is continually accessing stored body fat and you should not be hungry until your next meal. When you follow this approach, you will immediately notice that it is really worthwhile to use the protein powder instead of eating foods that will cause you to be mentally sluggish and perform poorly throughout the day.

Your physical activity levels determine how much protein powder you will need. If you walk about 15-20 minutes every day, you need only 1 teaspoon 2-4 times a day. If you work out daily for about 10-30 minutes, you'll need about 1 teaspoon 3-5 times daily. If you do weight training and jog, or work out more than 30 minutes daily, you will need 2 teaspoons 3-5 times daily.

Remember, it is not beneficial for you to consume too much protein at one time. Smaller amounts spread apart throughout the day have are far more effective at boosting HGH and IGF-1 levels and maintaining hormonal balance in our bodies.

Here's a summary of some of these simple anti-aging rules:

1   Always try to avoid age-accelerating foods: processed and cured meats, dairy foods, eggs, margarine, mayonnaise, sugar, artificial sweeteners, refined flours, coffee, salt, and sodas.

2   Emphasize age-reversing foods, especially the vegetables listed in Table 2. Visualize every meal containing at least half of these important foods.

3   Eat one or two large salads daily.

4   Season foods liberally with ginger, turmeric, mustards, and fresh or dried herbs.

5   Keep your intake of animal protein to a minimum. Never consume more animal protein than you can fit on the palm of your hand.

6   Drink herbal teas, sparkling waters with lemon or lime, filtered water, fresh grapefruit juice, and tomato juice.

7   Do not skip meals. Try to keep your meals about 5 hours apart. When you must skip a meal, always take your protein powder mixed with water or juice.

8   Do not eat late meals.

By following this diet plan and breaking bad dietary habits, you preserve your genetic blueprint, boost your levels of HGH and IGH-1 and consequently live your

70's, 80's, and 90's in excellent health. You decide how much you want to do and when you want to do it. After you experience what it is like to feel vibrant and young again, you will want to do more.

## KEY POINTS TO REMEMBER...

♦ The LII Anti-Aging diet plan is designed to boost the body's natural production of hormones and neurotransmitters while giving it superior antioxidant and alkaline-promoting foods that will contribute to maximum longevity.

♦ Eating age-accelerating foods, you will activate a multiplicity of age-accelerating mechanisms into motion that will eventually elevate your biological age well past your chronological age.

♦ The LII diet plan is designed to help you avoid the cyclic overeating and calorie-counting diets which will prevent you from functioning at peak capacity. Think about living to the age of 100 and still having the health you had when you were 30.

## WHAT YOU CAN DO NOW

♦ If dieting is hard for you, start with a transitional diet, slowly decreasing your intake of age-accelerating foods and increasing your intake of age-reversing foods. By doing so, you are now on the path of striving toward certain dietary goals.

♦ Try to meet these goals to the best of your ability without expecting too much, too fast. In time, as you feel younger, more vibrant and people comment about how great you look, you will be able to take each new step forward by eating more of the food choices outlined in this chapter.

So, go for it!

We are sure you'll be pleased with the results!

# CHAPTER 10

# LII LIFESTYLE MODIFICATION PROGRAM

One of the most important discoveries in aging research is that how you live and think contribute more to your ability to age successfully than genetics!

Even more importantly, lifestyle and attitude can even override your body's genetic programming to make you younger – or older. So rather than be a passive victim of genetics, you can now take control of how you age by following the principles outlined in this program. These principles will require some effort on your part, but this does not mean your life will suddenly become austere or deprived.

To the contrary, the people who practice these principles are people who lead fuller, happier and more satisfied lives than most!

Many people believe that the reason people are living longer than ever before is due to the advances in medical care. But research shows that medical care can only affect 10 percent of the factors that contribute to ill health…such as the eradication of a virus or bacteria, surgical removals or corrections and the alleviation of symptoms of various diseases.

Ninety percent of our health relies on habits over which doctors have no control such as smoking, stress, nutrition and exercise. Since you can control these habits, you actually have nine times more influence over your health and longevity than the medical profession. Preventing disease through a healthy lifestyle as suggested in this program is far more effective than treating it after it occurs.

The deterioration we see among the elderly is mistakenly taken for granted as a "normal" part of getting older. But many of these conditions truly are not normal at all. "Primary aging" such as slower reflexes, dimmer eyesight and decreased stamina are part of the primary aging process. However, many of the more serious afflictions – diabetes, Parkinson's disease, heart attacks – are called "secondary aging" and are not the direct results of aging, but of our own abuse of our bodies and ignorance about their needs.

Research into aging has clearly shown that secondary aging is NOT normal or inevitable. If you EXPECT some of these disorders to overtake you, now is the time to change your expectations and use this program, designed especially to help you do just that.

## PURPOSE IS ESSENTIAL TO SUCCESSFUL AGING

People who age successfully have a sense of purpose in their lives. In some cases it comes through work and their sense of what they are contributing to the business organization. Youthful individuals demonstrate a high degree of satisfaction with their jobs.

For others, purpose comes through their family and the sense that they are helping a spouse, children, or grandparents. Meaningful purpose may manifest in civic or neighborhood activities that make folks feel they're supporting the community. Many older people who stay young are often involved in volunteer work.

Whatever the source, people who age successfully have developed a sense they are needed, that their role in

146

life is important and when they retire at night, it is with the sense that the day was well spent.

## NUTRITIOUS EATING: A MUST FOR STAYING YOUNG

Another key characteristic of those who age successfully is their nutritious eating habits. These people eat regularly, usually at the same day each day. They do not skip meals and they refuse to cram their meals into a busy schedule. They seldom combine work with eating unless this is truly relaxing in itself.

Eating a nutritious breakfast is the most important meal investment of the day, Youthful adults are neither overweight or underweight. They eat age-reversing foods that strengthen the immune system and guard the body against the symptoms of premature aging. Their diet contains foods rich in vitamins, minerals and the essential and necessary fatty acid to promote healthy skin and hair, strong bones and mental alertness. These foods increase vitality and energy, help rid the body of toxins and speed the fat-burning process.

During the process of changing eating habits many individuals give in to social pressures and stop following the LII Anti-Aging Diet Plan. Ridicule from friends who may call you an "extremist" or a "health food nut" may cause some to surrender and subsequently consume excessive amounts of age-accelerating foods.

Giving in to social pressures often results in a retaliation of old symptoms and feelings of self-betrayal and self-denial. The excess consumption of sugar, caffeine, saturated fats, and simple carbohydrates causes symptoms—headaches, fatigue, irritability—that can only be alleviated by further addictive use of these substances. Rather than allowing yourself to get trapped in the vicious cycle of addiction and accelerated aging, remember how much better you felt when you ate more age-reversing foods.

Giving in to social pressures jeopardizes your body's delicate emotional and physical balance. There is something inherently wrong with friendships that produce social pressures and force a person to participate in destructive lifestyles. A real friend will not break your resolve to follow a health-promoting lifestyle.

Emotional symptoms may make it hard for us to stick to a healthy nutrition, diet, and exercise plan at times. Take a few moments to evaluate your mind-body connection. Rate the occurrence of each emotional symptom using the following scale:

0= NEVER 1 = OCCASIONALLY 2 = FREQUENTLY 3 = ALMOST ALWAYS

## A Self-Evaluation Of Your Emotional Status And Attitudes

___Difficult relationships

___Unable to relax

___Unable to forgive others

___Unable to forgive yourself

___Feel like a victim

___Unable to have a good time

___Low self-esteem

___Low self-confidence

___Find it difficult to love others or receive love

___Unresolved anger and bitterness

___Fearful

___Hide your true feelings

___Addictions: work, alcohol, caffeine, sugar, foods, sex, etc.

___Feel out of control

___Lonely or isolated

Now calculate your total score. If your score is in the range of 1-8, you have a mild emotional imbalance. If your score is in the range of 9-20, you may have a moderate to severe emotional imbalance.

People who score low on this test have the ability to manage stress. They know simple relaxation techniques. They have become expert at providing themselves with the tools they need to stay calm and collected and feel good about themselves. Some find a massage, a walk on the beach, daily exercise, or a long vacation helpful to unwind from stress. They recognize the symptoms of stress and find it easy to forgive and give unconditional love to people. They are aware of and responsive to their own bodies and minds.

When stress begins to harm them they take affirmative action. By changing their attitudes about life and stress, these individuals use their stress to stay young. By dealing with it creatively, they slowly improve their work, their personal skills and relationships.

These individuals are not harsh, unreasoning, punishing, or unforgiving. They have learned to develop a genuine interest in their health and well being. The are motivated by their progress and fail to get discouraged from their occasional setbacks.

Most importantly, they have the strength, courage

and awareness to continue with their quest for a long, healthy life.

If we view our mistakes as learning experiences, we can see the positive aspects of every life experience. Difficulties and setbacks are seen as challenges to overcome.

Come to view adversity as a challenge and try to be creative in problem solving. Youthful people are optimistic and unafraid to take risks. Their optimism allows them to be unafraid of failure.

Those who stay young have a sense of humor about life and themselves. They are able to take life lightly, to see the grand comedy in it all. They can laugh at their own flaws and mistakes. Most importantly, they know how to play, smile and laugh. They are open, loving, enthusiastic and fun. They are responsible, informed and committed.

## INTEGRATING RIGHT AND LEFT BRAIN WITH HEMI-SYNC

The Monroe Institute of Faber, Virginia has developed a powerful stress-relief and cognitive enhancement approach that is based on integrating the right and left brain. The process that the institute has developed is known as Hemi-Sync, an abbreviation of Hemispheric Synchronization.[1,2]

What is truly amazing about the Hemi-Sync process is that it produces whole brain coherence—a state of mental functioning that dramatically helps us to meet the challenges of stress and function at a higher state of mental activity. The process uses frequencies that stimulate whole body functioning in the quantic domain.

Once an individual is trained with these frequencies, learning to reproduce them at will, without the audio stimulation becomes possible.

These frequencies are in the beta, alpha, theta, delta, and other ranges; that is, from 30 Hz to 0.5 Hz. When combined in certain sequences these can stimulate greater concentration, deep relaxation, and enhanced learning. The result: the production of a highly focused, coherent and productive mind-brain state.

These mind-brain exercises promise to increase intellectual capacity while sharpening intuitive senses and physical abilities. Stress-related conditions, anxiety, tension and pain are relieved without drug-induced side effects or addictions.

If you are interested in thinking more clearly, improving your memory, and freeing yourself from fear, the Monroe in-home training system may be your answer. Full details of all Monroe Institute products as well as Hemi-Sync training tapes are available by writing to LII.

Here is one immediately available, simple technique to start using now from the Monroe Institute: Visualize a rapidly running river turning a bend and coming back into itself so as to create a circle. Make the river overflow itself so that the inside of the circle floods and creates a perfectly smooth lake. Now, imagine yourself in this watery, mirror-like calm with a slight smile!

This technique allows you to take your anger, neutralize and dissociate it, replacing it with an opposite emotion. It also allows you to see that you are the one who decides whether to let the "present situation" affect you or let it go by. In essence, you are solely responsible for your own reactions, maybe not the situation, but certainly how the situation effects you!

151

## SOUND HEALING

Sound can also be used as a form of healing. Like a unique fingerprint our body develops an electromagnetic pattern of energies with advancing age. This pattern reflects itself through many body systems including the voice. The Chinese knew the sound of the voice of a person could be used to diagnose energetic disharmonics.

Dr. Marcellus Walker and Christina Walker, RN, MA use a computer-based system which analyzes the harmonic stresses of the voice and correlates these with a person's health issues and deficiency states. This unique system of therapy reverberates a harmonic frequency that is intended to strengthen the deficiencies of the body. For further information, see APPENDIX C.

## EXERCISE PROGRAM KEY FOR THOSE WHO STAY YOUNG

Youthful adults exercise at least three or more times a week. They choose exercises that are appropriate for the needs of their body, that will work to keep them fit, strong and flexible. In most cases, that means they stay on a regular program of aerobic exercise such as walking, swimming, bicycling or moderate jogging.

These exercises reinforce the immune system and strengthen the cardiovascular system. These exercises help improve the body's oxygen capacity so nutrients can be carried through as toxins are carried out. They increase flexibility, coordination, reflex responses and other skills.

People who stay young are committed to their exercise program and rarely miss a workout. In fact, they all say that exercise is enjoyable, energizing as well as being their favorite part of the day. Regular exercise is a characteristic of the youthful 40 year olds as well as the youthful 80 year olds - exercise has no age limit.

The normal wear and tear of aging can cause structural disorders and a lack of flexibility in joints and muscles. These biomarkers of the aging process respond to exercise, stretching, and relaxation techniques—all things you can control.

There are five anti-aging breathing and stretching exercises that activate the powerful anti-aging centers of the body. These exercises improve Level 1 biomarkers (increased flexibility in joints, improved pulmonary function, etc.) and oxygenate body tissues while allowing it to get rid of excessive acidity (pH-balancing effects).

In addition, these exercises relax the nervous system, leaving us in a calm mental state. Every position sends a molecular message to the core centers of our cellular environment and excites different molecular functions of our cellular soup. These different positions activate acupuncture points and vital energy centers of the body, and radically diminish the chance that you'll be grimacing with pain with advancing age.

Be sure to take a series of deep breaths before and after each positional exercise. You can start these amazing exercises in the following manner:

1    While standing erect with your arms outstretched, horizontal with your shoulders, roll your head around from left to right 2-12 times. If you placed a clock on the floor face up, you would turn clockwise. Start with only two complete rotations, then each week increase one rotation until you

are able to do 12 complete rotations without getting dizzy or losing your balance. Finally, Take 6 deep breaths.

2    While laying flat on your back on an exercise mat or rug, place your hands flat down alongside your hips. Slowly raise your legs without bending your knees. Set a goal to eventually raise your legs until they are straight up. Take 6 deep breaths.

3    While kneeling on the rug, place your hands on your thighs and lean forward as far as possible while resting your chin on your chest. Now lean backwards while lifting your head as far as it will go. Repeat this process 2-6 times. Take 6 deep breaths.

4    While sitting on the rug, stretch your feet out in front of you while keeping your hands flat down. Now raise your body while bending your knees so that your legs, from the knees down, are straight up and down. In this position, your arms, too, will be straight up and down, while the body, from the shoulders to the knees, will be horizontal. Alternate between stretching and relaxing in a sitting position. Take 6 deep breaths.

5    Place both hands on the floor about two feet apart like you are preparing to do a pushup. Then, push the body, especially the hips, up as far as possible, rising on the toes and hands. Next, allow the body to slowly come down to a sagging position letting your head drop down slowly. Then, conclude these exercises with a series of deep breaths.

Twenty minutes of walking before you eat breakfast, helps to reset your metabolic rate, allowing you to burn off excessive calories in fats consumed from the day before. Most importantly, the combination of the five stretching and breathing exercises (five-ten minutes) with twenty minutes of early morning walking in a fasting state of metabolism, enhances HGH levels and speeds up the rate of nutrient delivery to your cellular soup.

Before you start any exercise program, be sure to engage in the five anti-aging stretch postures. Running, walking, treadmill running, weight-training and using a stationary bike before you eat breakfast are great ways to boost HGH activity. If you exercise after breakfast, the release of HGH is minimal.

**CAUTION: Do not start an exercise program without <u>first consulting your family physician.</u>**

POINTS TO REMEMBER...

♦ The key to staying young is to adopt a healthy lifestyle and change old destructive beliefs and attitudes that damage your mental and physical health.

♦ By eliminating bad habits, you have nine times more influence over your health than the medical profession.

♦ Start today to form a new view of your potential life span and be optimistic about lowering your current biological age. This new belief system will have a positive impact on your biological age.

## WHAT YOU CAN DO NOW

♦ Think positive and view your mistakes as learning experiences.

♦ View difficulties and setbacks as challenges to overcome.

♦ Exercise daily and practice the five anti-aging stretching techniques outlined in this chapter.

# CHAPTER 11

# FUTURE DIRECTIONS FOR ANTI-AGING MEDICINE

For as long as scientists have studied aging, they have nurtured the dream of being able to stop genes from mutating and going bad. Certain genes act as the cell's director of damage control by producing protective proteins that shield our genetic blueprint from damage. But our toxic environment—cigarette smoke, ionizing radiation, chemical carcinogens, chemotherapy drugs—damages these protective genes.

Once a protective gene is mutated, it starts churning out mutant proteins and no longer is capable of producing necessary protective proteins. Mutant proteins form molecular nets that degrade and choke off many cellular functions which then activate a cell's suicide program.

This book has described a newly emerging system of the health care based on a the concept of preserving the integrity of the living cell's genes. These profound discoveries offer us unlimited possibilities for life extension. Helping you to understand how to protect the elegant genetic system that nature has engineered, is the primary goal of this book. Keeping our cells on the path of normalcy by revitalizing our cellular soup will prevent cells from dying faster than they renew—the primary cause of premature aging.

Because of the rising number of age-related disorders, a way of seeing ourselves as "whole men or women" becomes indispensable. This concept of

Quantum Nutrition owes its origins to the medical practices of ancient and traditional cultures where a valuable legacy of thousands of years of empirical experience provides powerful therapeutic guidelines.

During the past three decades, progress in understanding how our bodies react to the world around us has accelerated significantly. The biological and physiological foundations for these growling regulatory abilities promise natural approaches to enhancing the functional status of the neuroendocrine system, preserving the genetic blueprint, and extending the life span.

One thing is certain: Lifestyle, not heredity, most influences our chances of avoiding age-related illnesses. The message is loud and clear: If we want to live longer and healthier we have to alter our lifestyles. If we wait until we have a medical crisis, it may be too late…and we will not be alive to take advantage of the new, exciting discoveries that will allow us to extend our lives to 100 and beyond.

Orthodox medicine has provided many tools for helping humans who are suffering from "crisis" symptoms and has provided doctors with information and knowledge to diagnose these "crisis" states of illness and successfully treat them medically.

These efforts, which deserve full recognition, consist of very specialized techniques for evaluating various parts of the whole human organism. However, it must always be remembered that the whole body is greater than the sum of its parts. Age-related illness will never be fully understood by the use of inanimate methods of exact scientific research concerned only with separate aspects of the whole body. For this reason, anti-aging medical approaches, scans or views the entire organism—from atoms to molecules to cells to organs and their systems—as advanced methods are used to preserve the genetic integrity of the entire body.

The components and electromagnetic nature of the genetic realm of biomolecular functioning can be understood rationally by means of multidisciplinary knowledge and logic. If one accepts only what is measurable and comprehensible as real, then the true nature of age-related illnesses may never be fully addressed and compensated for by anti-aging physicians of the future.

As research on anti-aging medicine continues, more evidence will uncover additional therapeutic measures that focus on logical and efficient ways of showing incontrovertibly that regulatory activities of the body can be tuned into awe-inspiring ways, stimulating the miraculous healing systems of total body rejuvenation. The extensive information now available indicates that aging is the end result of a defective chain of events. Each link in the chain of events must be strengthened, balanced and synchronized for true health and healing to take place.

With this new information about the nature of human aging available, science becomes challenged and public pressure on science and medicine increases. These pressures on the scientific community stimulate them to perform more relevantly to human needs and present demands.

The past few decades have seen a remarkable reversal of medicine's domination over ideas of how to treat illness and diagnose age-related illnesses. These illuminated anti-aging experts share a new vision of the human body and its untapped healing potential. As a result they will continue to witness how preserving the genetic blueprint is extending and improving the quality of life.

## NEW TECHNOLOGIES ON THE HORIZON

Technical development in the field of anti-aging medicine has brought not only blessings but progress to mankind. Science has discovered ways to reverse aging that are within reach for all of us. Stopping the body's aging clock and celebrating our 100th, 200th, and even 300th birthday is on the not-to-distant horizon for anti-aging scientists.

LII is at the forefront of this new era. Our research and program has already resulted in slowing down this aging clock. Now we are on the verge of developing hormonal pacemaker devices and other technologies that turn back the aging clock, allowing us to maintain the youthful vitality of a twenty-year-old. Once this has been accomplished, the body will have the amazing ability to continually regenerate itself by replacing molecules, cells, and tissues at optimal levels.

In the future, the fundamental processes of aging will be explored more fully. Scientists have already unraveled many of the complex forces involved in the aging process. On the horizon are the following exciting prospects for extending longevity:[1-11]

♦ GENETIC TELOMERE-BASED RESEARCH - Telomeres— sequences of nucleic acids extending from the ends of a chromosome—are providing new insights into the enzyme telomerase which stimulates the repair and replacement in telomeres as we age. When telomeres are damaged, the cell ages and dies. New exciting possibilities are now being explored by pharmaceutical companies to devise drugs that will target and destroy telemorase in cancer cells without disrupting the normal function of healthy cells. Another decade of telomere research should also help to reveal how drug inhibitors of telomerase can selectively activate the telomerase in normal cells while simultaneously blocking this enzymes activity in cancer cells.

♦ GENETIC-P53 RESEARCH - A gene called p53—the cell's most elegant defender—stops tumors before they grow. Scientists are discovering ways to stop aging cells from heading down the path toward cancer. Since p53 acts as the cell's director of damage control, scientists are currently exploring ways to tap into nature's elegant system of controlling aging at the genetic level.

♦ PHYTOCHEMICAL RESEARCH - Data emerging from many university laboratories underscores the role for phytochemicals found in fruits, vegetables and grains as ways to protect and preserve our genetic blueprint from free-radicals and environmental toxins. LII has already incorporated this data into our diet and nutritional plan. However, future studies may reveal ways to extract more powerful antioxidant agents from plants.

♦ HORMONAL PRECURSOR RESEARCH - The most exciting prospects currently are secretagogues for boosting HGH and IGF-1 levels. LII has developed the first nutritional secretagogue-peptide formulation—and the clinical results are impressive! In addition, LII has developed and researched a hormone precursor formulation with PREG and DHEA designed to boost many anti-aging functions of the body. Precursor-based formulations, energized by Quantum Nutrition, translate into the reality of allowing the body to produce its own hormones...naturally. Currently, LII is working on developing transdermal and other novel approaches for delivering hormones naturally to various cells of the body.

♦ PHARMACEUTICAL-BASED RESEARCH - Numerous anti-aging medicines are being developed and should available sometime in the next decade. In the interim, **Table 5** in the Appendix provides you with a list of anti-aging hormones and precursors, medicines, and nutrients currently available at pharmacies, health food stores, and through mail order.

## ADVANCED DIAGNOSTICS: THE BIOMARKER MATRIX PROTOCOL

The Biomarker Matrix Protocol is the most advanced and accurate way yet to determine the body's biological age and not its chronological age. These biomarkers are also predictive of the individual's risk for developing age-related disorders. Biomarkers are enzymes, skin cells and biochemicals produced by the body. These Biomarkers help to clearly identify the signs of accelerated aging long before pathology is observed.

The LII Biomarker Matrix Protocol consists of four levels of assessment:

**Level 1** - Biomarkers begin with the effects of aging on the physiological level or overall functioning of the client. Basic "surface indicators" include:

-Muscle Mass/Body Fat Ratio

-Flexibility

-Aerobic Capacity

-Bone Density

-Tactile Response Time

-Forced Expiatory Volume

-Visual and Auditory Tests

**Level 2** - Biomarkers evaluate aging at the cellular level. This includes a skin biopsy of areas of the body not exposed to the sun but which show histological evidence of aging in the skin. This analysis may include evaluation of:

-Basement membrane changes

-Epidermal turnover rates.

-Collagen ratios

-Sebaceous gland architecture

-Microvascular changes

-Elastic fiber content

**Level 3** - Biomarkers evaluate aging on the molecular level. This is done by analyzing biochemical assays of various serum extractions including:

-Key biomarker hormones including DHEA, HGH, and thyroid hormone

-Melatonin

-Cellular CoEnzyme Q10

-Insulin sensitivity & heat shock proteins

-Oncogene surveys, Elongation Factor 1

**Level 4** - Biomarkers evaluate aging on the chromosomal level. This analysis utilizes the latest technology in gene therapy and examines gene structure which includes length, telomere position, and DNA strand breakage rates. A number of other genetic tests included in level 4 studies help to evaluate the aging process at its origin, the genetic cellular level.

**Level 5** - Biomarkers evaluate aging on the electromagnetic level. This analysis uses advanced German medical diagnostic systems to measure deficits in the body's energy field and ascertain more about how Quantum Nutrition can counteract the aging process.

As we explore the frontiers of anti-aging medicine, we learn that our cellular soup— governed by the laws of quantum physics—can be improved to the point of lowering our biological age and extending our life span. For the first time in the history of medicine we are on the verge of understanding the mysteries of life at the molecular level. Quantum energies influence and control molecules into precise, beautiful, powerful organic compounds: genes.

The quantum dimension of life and human functioning can widen our horizons, enlarge our comprehension of the aging process, and help us grasp the path of Anti-Aging Medicine into the 21st century.

Understanding anti-aging therapeutics at the quantum level of Nature will allow physicians of the future to trigger powerful anti-aging response at the sub-atomic domain of human functioning and also understand the mysterious breakdowns in human functioning that occur at the genetic level as we age. Every stage of life occurs according to DNA's timetable.

What makes DNA operate in this manner?

Leading quantum physicists have documented the fact that DNA operates in the quantum level of Nature. As with all quantum events, the super-genius of DNA, is not limited solely to the chemical or molecular domain of human functioning. At the quantum level of functioning, DNA manages to perform super feats of regulating all that happens in our bodies. True solutions to premature aging will ultimately come from scientists and physicians that address this hidden world of unseen and life-governing energies. By using hormone precursors, Quantum Nutrition and anti-aging foods, LII's Anti-Aging Plan attempts to protect and preserve the multiplicity of powerful DNA functions.

The LII Anti-Aging Plan brings together research from many scientific disciplines to demonstrate that the controlling the aging process means changing the basic patterns that design our physiology—with the potential to defeat age-associated diseases and even aging itself.

### POINTS TO REMEMBER...

♦ For you to experience true health and healing, each link in the body's age-related chain of events must be strengthened, balanced, and synchronized.

- ◆ Lifestyle, not heredity influences your chances of avoiding age-related diseases.

- ◆ Following the LII Anti-Aging Plan will take you one step closer to a longer, healthier life.

- ◆ All your years of hard work can be best rewarded with good health. By following the LII Anti-Aging Plan you can reap this reward.

### WHAT YOU CAN DO NOW

- ◆ Review the POINTS TO REMEMBER sections at the end of each chapter.

- ◆ Take a long, honest look at your diet. What you eat—or abstain from eating—has a lot to do with premature aging. It is more urgent than ever for you to take charge now of both the quantity and quality of the food you eat.

- ◆ Take a good look at your environment. Try to eliminate toxic chemicals in your home or workplace that are known to target your genetic blueprint (see APPENDIX A).

### TABLE 5: ANTI-AGING HORMONES, HORMONE PRECURSORS, AND MEDICINES

| HORMONES | EFFECTS |
|---|---|
| **DHEA** energizes, may improve memory and libido, helps to reduce body fat, anti-stress, boosts immunity. | |
| **PREGNENOLONE** is a precursor to all steroid hormones, may enhance memory and concentration. | |

166

**HGH** helps to strengthen the heart and muscles, burns fat, accelerates repair and regeneration.

**IGF-1** enhances protein synthesis and repair functions.

**Melatonin** may enhance sexual vigor, antioxidant, anti-stress effects, may restore normal sleep patterns and cure jet lag.

**Thyroid Hormone** maintains body temperature and metabolic rate, enhances many body functions.

**Estrogen** may enhance mood and sexual function, may enhance skin quality and prevent heart, bone, and colon disease.

**Testosterone** enhances sex drive, may protect against heart and bone disorders, builds muscle, lowers cholesterol.

**Progesterone** boosts the action of estrogen, potential treatment for cancer and nerve disease.

**Estriol** anti-cancer, anti-cyst, anti-tumor part of the tri-estrogen complex.

HORMONE PRECURSORS     FUNCTION

**PREGURSEX** Fatty acid esters of PREG and DHEA to augment the formation of progesterone, testosterone, cortisol, estrogen, and other steroid hormones.

**EndoSync** Cholesterol-free sources of precursors for anti-inflammatory ecosanoid hormones.

**SynchroPower** Secretagogue-peptides for enhancement of HGH and IGF-1 and amino acid analogue hormones.

**NeuroSync** Neurohormone precursors and precursors for the formation of neurotransmitters.

PHARMACEUTICAL DRUGS    FUNCTION

**Metformin** is an anti-diabetic drug that reduces insulin levels and lowers cholesterol.

**Deprenyl** used in the treatment of Parkinson's disease and Alzheimer's diseases has been found to boost nervous system transmitters and restore nervous system sensitivity causing mental stimulation and increased alertness.

**Piracetam** is a drug found to increase cognitive abilities, especially memory and attention span in geriatric patients. It works by stimulating cellular energy cycles and also enhances the body's ability to manufacture proteins and phospholipids (fat molecules that protect the cell membrane and neurons).

**Hydergine** is prescribed for age-related decline in mental capacity to help reverse memory loss and to preserve brain functioning.

**GHB (gamma hydroxylbutyrate)** is a naturally occurring compound found in every cell of the body. It functions as a precursor to a neurotransmitter called GABA (gamma-aminobutyric acid) involved in the regulation of the pituitary gland. As a result of its direct action on the pituitary gland, many researchers feel it is a potent stimulator of HGH. However, severe liver toxicity, nausea, vomiting, loss of consciousness, tremors, respiratory disorder, seizures, and coma may occur with this drug.

**5 HTP (5-hydroxyltryptophan)** represents the most powerful natural approach to replacing common anti-anxiety and anti-depression medications. 5-HTP is a precursor to serotonin which is a precursor to melatonin. Studies have shown it to be clinically effective in individuals suffering from anxiety, depression, and irritability of the nervous system.

**Gerovital H3** developed by Ana Aslan, M.D., improves memory and energy levels and has a rejuvenating effect at the cell level.

# APPENDIX A:
## COMMON AGE-ACCELERATING ADDITIVES

**Artificial colorings** are synthetic chemicals that do not occur in nature. Colorings are not always listed by name on labels. However, colorings are used almost solely in age-promoting foods of low nutritional value (candy, soda pop, gelatin desserts, etc.).

**Blue No. 1** - Found in beverages, candy, and some baked goods. May be carcinogenic.

**Blue No. 2** - Artificial coloring in pet food, beverages, and candy. May be carcinogenic.

**Citrus Red No. 2** - Artificial coloring found in the skin of some Florida oranges. Although this is a proven carcinogenic coloring, this dye does not seep through the orange skin into the pulp.

**Green No. 3** - Artificial coloring in candy, and some beverages. May cause bladder cancer.

**Red No. 3** - Found in cherries in fruit cocktail, candy, and some baked goods. Causes thyroid tumors in rats.

**Yellow No. 6** - Found in beverages, sausage, baked goods, candy and gelatin. This dye causes tumors of the adrenal gland and kidney and is contaminated with cancer-causing impurities.

**Brominated vegetable oil (BVO)** - Used as an emulsifier, clouding agent in soft drinks. May be carcinogenic.

**Butylated Hydroxyanisole (BHA)** - found in cereals, chewing gum, potato chips, and vegetable oils. Causes cancer in rats.

**Caffeine** - found in stimulant, coffee, tea, cocoa (natural), soft drinks (additive). Caffeine may throw hormones out of balance and triggers accelerated molecular aging.

**Propyl Gallate** - found in vegetable oils, meat products, potato sticks, chicken soup base, and chewing gum. May cause cancer.

**Quinine** - found in flavoring, tonic water, quinine water, and bitter lemon. May be carcinogenic.

**Saccharin** - Used as synthetic sweetener in "diet" products. The FDA proposed that saccharin be banned, because of repeated evidence that it causes cancer.

**Salt (sodium chloride)** - Found in flavoring, most processed foods, soup, potato chips, and crackers. Disturbs the balance of our cellular soup. Use lightly or replace with sea salt.

**Sodium Nitrate, sodium nitrate** - A preservative found in bacon, ham, frankfurters, luncheon meats, smoked fish, and corned beef. Leads to formation of small amounts of potent cancer-causing chemicals (nitrosamines).

**Sugar (sucrose)** - Used as a sweetener. Found in table sugar and sweetened foods. Disturbs hormonal and chemical balance of cellular soup.

**Sulfur dioxide, Sodium Bisulfite** - Found in bleach dried fruit, wine and processed potatoes. Has already caused seven deaths and may be carcinogenic.

# APPENDIX B:
## INSTRUCTIONS FOR LII BIOMARKER SELF-TEST

Test I: *PERCENT BODY FAT* = 15% Men 22% Females
IDEAL PERCENT BODY FAT: To determine your body fat levels, stand naked in front of a mirror. If you're a male or female and can clearly see your abdominal muscles, you are at the ideal percent of body fat.

BORDERLINE PERCENT BODY FAT: If you're a male and cannot see your abdominal muscles but have no "love handles," you're at 15 percent body fat. If you are a female and have no "cellulite," you are approximately at 22 percent body fat.

ABNORMAL PERCENT BODY FAT: If you are a male and have "love handles," or a female with cellulite you have excessive body fat.

*WEIGHT*
Check your weight against the following chart. Subtract your weight from the ideal anti-aging weights and record the difference on your test sheet.

## MEN

| HEIGHT | SMALL FRAME | MEDIUM FRAME | LARGE FRAME |
|--------|-------------|--------------|-------------|
| 5' 1"  | 107-115     | 113-124      | 121-136     |
| 5' 2"  | 110-118     | 116-128      | 124-148     |
| 5' 3"  | 113-121     | 119-131      | 127-143     |
| 5' 4"  | 116-124     | 122-134      | 131-147     |
| 5' 5"  | 119-128     | 125-138      | 133-151     |
| 5' 6"  | 123-132     | 129-142      | 137-156     |
| 5' 7"  | 127-136     | 125-138      | 133-151     |
| 5' 8"  | 131-140     | 137-151      | 146-156     |
| 5' 9"  | 135-145     | 141-155      | 150-169     |
| 5' 10" | 139-149     | 145-160      | 154-174     |

## MEN (CONTINUED):

| HEIGHT | SMALL FRAME | MEDIUM FRAME | LARGE FRAME |
|---|---|---|---|
| 5' 11" | 143-153 | 149-165 | 159-179 |
| 6' | 147-157 | 153-170 | 163-187 |
| 6' 1" | 151-162 | 157-175 | 168-189 |
| 6' 2" | 155-166 | 162-180 | 173-194 |
| 6' 3" | 159-170 | 167-185 | 177-199 |

## WOMEN

| HEIGHT | SMALL FRAME | MEDIUM FRAME | LARGE FRAME |
|---|---|---|---|
| 4' 9" | 89-95 | 93-104 | 101-116 |
| 4' 10" | 91-98 | 95-107 | 103-119 |
| 4' 11" | 93-101 | 98-110 | 106-122 |
| 5' | 96-104 | 101-113 | 109-125 |
| 5' 1" | 99-107 | 104-116 | 112-128 |
| 5' 2" | 102-110 | 107-119 | 115-131 |
| 5' 3" | 105-113 | 110-123 | 118-135 |
| 5' 4" | 108-116 | 113-127 | 122-139 |
| 5' 5" | 111-120 | 117-132 | 126-143 |
| 5' 6" | 115-124 | 121-136 | 130-147 |
| 5' 7" | 119-128 | 125-140 | 134-151 |
| 5' 8" | 123-132 | 129-144 | 138-155 |
| 5' 9" | 127-137 | 133-148 | 142-160 |
| 5' 10" | 131-141 | 137-152 | 146-165 |
| 5' 11" | 135-145 | 141-156 | 150-170 |

*SKIN ELASTICITY TEST*:

Pinch the skin on the back of your hand between the thumb and forefinger for 5 seconds. Time how long it takes the skin to flatten out completely. If it takes 5 seconds or more, you have an abnormal skin elasticity test.

*STATIC BALANCE TEST*: To do this test, stand on a hard surface (not a rug) while keeping both feet (no shoes) flat on the ground. To be on the safe side, have a friend standing by to catch you in case you start to fall over. Close your eyes and lift your foot about six inches off the ground. Lift your left foot if you are right-handed and your right foot if you are left-handed. Have your friend time how long you can do this without opening your eyes or moving your foot to avoid falling over. Repeat this test three times and compute the average time that you can stand one-legged with your eyes closed. If you can stand for 30 seconds or more without falling or opening your eyes, you have a normal test score. Less than 30 seconds constitutes an abnormal static balance test.

# APPENDIX C:
## ANTI-AGING RESOURCES

The American Academy of Anti-Aging Medicine (A4M) is the first clinical society of physicians and researchers to address the phenomenon of human aging as a treatable medical condition. Its mission is to identify, disseminate and publicize information on treatment options that stabilize and forestall the deleterious effects of aging. To this end, A4M is dedicated to bringing a new paradigm to health-care practitioners around the world. For further information, write to A4M at 90 South Cascade, Colorado Springs, CO 80903 or World Health Network - http://www.worldhealth.net

The Longevity Institute International (LII), founded by Vincent C. Giampapa, M.D. in 1996, is the first accredited scientific anti-aging treatment and diagnostic center in the world. It is a completely unique medical, health and fitness research organization which employs revolutionary techniques designed to measure, treat and retard the aging process. For further information, write LII at 89 Valley Road, Montclair, NJ 07042 or call 201-746-3535.

### LII AND A4M ANTI-AGING BOOKS:

*Grow Young with HGH* by Dr. Ronald Klatz with Carol Kahn, Harper-Collins Publisher, 1997.

*Stopping the Clock* by Dr. Ron Klatz and Dr. Bob Goldman, Keats Publishing, 1996.

*Miracle Hormones...Naturally* by Dr. Paul Yanick, Jr. and Vincent C. Giampapa, M.D., Kensington Publishing, 1997.

*BioRegulation, Regeneration, and LifeSpan Extension,* Dr. Paul Yanick, Jr., Ph.D. LII, 1995.

*Advances in Anti-Aging Medicine,* edited by Dr. Ron Klatz, Mary Ann Liebert, Inc. Publishers, 1995.

*The Science of Anti-Aging Medicine,* edited by Dr. Ron Klatz and Dr. Bob Goldman, A4M, 1996.

*Anti-Aging Secrets* by Dr. Ron Klatz and Dr. Bob Goldman, A4M, 1996.

**ALTERNATIVE HEALING THROUGH SOUND:**
Sound Healing by Christina Walker, RN, MA, 1855 Fair Avenue, Honesdale, PA 18431, Phone #1-888-AntiAGE.

# APPENDIX D:
## SOURCES FOR SUPERIOR
## ANTI-AGING NUTRITIONAL PRODUCTS

*A.C. Grace Company*- A superior and pure form of unesterified Vitamin E
1100 Quit Man Road
Big Sandy, TX 75755
903-636-4368

*Longevity Institute International* - Exclusive source for Quantum Nutritional products: SynchroPower™, EndoSync™, PREGURSEX™, SYNCHROX™, and the LII Oral Supplement Program.
89 Valley Road,
Montclair, NJ 07042
201-746-3535

*Nutraceutics* - Source of NeuroSync™ and other superior hormone precursor products.
600 Fairway Drive, Suite 105
Deerfield Beach, FL 33441
1-800-391-0114

*Pacific Research Laboratories* - Source of pure, superior, bioenergetic nutritional and herbal products.
1010 Crenshaw Blvd., Suite 250
Torrance, CA 90501
310-787-8751

# DR. PAUL YANICK, JR., PH.D.
## LECTURE PRESENTATIONS

With energy born of confidence, optimism, and scientific efficiently, Dr. Paul Yanick, Jr., challenges, motivates, and inspires people to tap into the awe of their body's marvelous self-healing and self-regenerating capacities—by preserving their genetic blueprint. He shares with his audience up-to-date information on how achieving *Quantum Longevity* is possible by activating anti-aging responses where aging begins—at the quantum or genetic domain of life. For the first time, he presents an anti-aging plan as a clinically effective method of preserving the body's genetic blueprint and activating youthful levels of hormones. As medical research director of the prestigious *Longevity Institute International (LII)*, Dr. Yanick presents cutting edge research that shows it is possible to live to 100 and beyond. . . without the frailties of old age.

Dr. Yanick knows the anguish and frustration of being told that he had fatal kidney and adrenal disease at the age of 20. Almost 3 decades ago he was given a year to live by leading medical experts. He has discovered secrets to longevity and is eager to share his experiences and knowledge with others. Dr. Yanick is a leader in the field of anti-aging medicine. His audience will learn the full story about how to put the brakes on aging with natural hormone therapies as he presents an exciting new wave of biotechnology and chemistry that enhances the body's production of youth-generating hormones—so the signs of old age may begin to fade.

## SUBJECT OPTIONS FOR A HEALTH LECTURE PRESENTATION

♦ Strategies for boosting natural hormone production without costly hormone injections and pills

♦ How to turn back the body's biological aging clock

♦ Male Menopause, DHEA and Testosterone

♦ Female Hormones: Balancing Progesterone, Estrogen, and Testosterone

♦ Miracle Hormones. . . Naturally

♦ Pregnenolone: The Missing Link in Anti-aging therapies

♦ NeuroNutrition: Nutrients that put the brakes on brain aging

♦ Secrets for staying young and vibrant

♦ NeuroNutrition: Tinnitus Relief

♦ Regenerating Hormone Therapies: DHEA, HGH, Pregnenolone, Testosterone and more!

Dr. Yanick offers cutting edge breakthroughs that go way beyond explaining isolated hormone disorders and provides individuals with a whole world of new and exciting possibilities for life span extension.

For information regarding Dr. Yanick's presentations and booking schedule, please contact Michael Goldman, P.O. Box 651, Cardiff, CA or call 619-753-6614 or FAX 619-753-6733.

# Text Footnotes:

## Chapter 1:

1.  Klatz, R. *Advances in Anti-Aging Medicine*, Vol. 1., New York: Mary Ann Liebert, Inc. Publishers, 1995.

2.  Dollins, A.B, Wurtman, R.J. & Deng, M. H. *Proc. netn. Acad. Sci.* U.S.A. 91. 1824-1828; 1994.

3.  Pierpaoli, W., and Lesnikov, V.A. The pineal aging clock. Evidence, models, mechanisms, interventions. *Ann N Y Acad Sci* 719:461-73; 1994.

4.  Huether, G. Melatonin synthesis in the gastrointestinal tract and the impact of nutritional factors on circulating Melatonin. *Annals NY Academy Sciences* 719:146-157; 1994.

5.  Cenacchi T, Bertoldin T, Farina C, Fiori MG, Crepaldi G. Cognitive decline in the elderly: A Double-blind, Placebo-controlled multicenter study on efficacy of phosphatidylserine administration. *Aging* (ITALY) 5:123-133: 1993.

6.  Yanick, P. *Bioregulation, Regeneration and Lifespan Extension*. Yanick, Inc. 1994.

7.  Morales, A.J., Nolan, J.N., Nelson, J.C., Yen, S.S. Effect of replacement dose of Dehydroepi-androsterone in men and women of advancing age. *J Clin Endocrinol Metab* 78: 1360-1367, 1994.

8.  Belanger, A., Candas, B., DuPont, A. et al. Changes in Serum concentrations of conjugated and unconjugated steroids in 40 to 80 year old men. *J Clin Endocrinol Metab* 79: 1086-1090, 1994.

9. Auernhammer, C.J., et al. "Effect of growth hormone and insulin-like growth factor I on the immune system," *Eur. J. Endocrinol.* 133:635-45, 1995.

10. Walford, R. "the Clinical Promise of Diet Restriction," *Geriatrics* 45 81-83, 86-87; 1990.

11. Walford, Roy L. *The One Hundred and Twenty Year Diet: How to double your vital years.* Simon & Schuster, NY, 1987.

## CHAPTER 3:

1. Stinnett, J.D. *Nutrition and the Immune Response,* CRC Press, Inc., Boca Raton, Florida, 1983.

2. Gill, G.V. et al., *Journal of Neurology, Neurosurgery, and Psychiatry,* Vol. 45, P. 861, 1982.

3. Ginter, E. *World Review of Nutrition and Dietetics,* Vol. 33, P. 104, 1979.

4. *Journal of the American Medical Association,* NIH, Vol. 253, P. 2080, April 12, 1985.

5. Quillin, P. "The Role of Nutrition in Cancer Treatment" *Health Counselor,* Vol. 4, No. 6.

6. Quillin, P. *Healing Nutrients,* Contemporary Books, Chicago, Illinois, pp. 43-52, 1987.

7. Sempos, C.T. et al., *Journal of the American Dietetic Association,* Vol. 81, P. 35, July 1982.

8. Schroeder, H. *American Journal of Clinical Nutrition,* Vol. 24, p. 562, May 1971.

9. Stinnett, J.D. et al. (eds.), "Proteins and Amino Acids- Prospects for Nutritional Therapy in Infection," *Relevance of Nutrition to Sepis*, Ross Laboratories, Columbia, Ohio, 1982.

10. *New England Journal of Medicine*, Vol. 243, pp. 617-621, 1984.

11. *Healthy People*, U.S. Department of Health, Education and Welfare, U.S. Government Printing Office, 79-55071, Washington D.C., p. 101, 1979.

12. Geissler, C. et al., *American Journal of Clinical Nutrition*, Vol. 31, 1978, p. 667; Vol. 39, p. 478, March 1984.

**CHAPTER 4:**

1. Lonsdale, D. "Free Oxygen Radicals and Disease," 1986/A Year in Nutritional Medicine Monograph, Keats Publishing, Inc. New Canaan, Conn., pp. 5-6, 1986.

2. Pryor, W.A. "Free radical biology: Xenobiotics, cancer," Annals N.Y. Academy of Sciences, 393:2-5, 1992.

3. Bland, J. "The Nutritional Effects of Free Radical Pathology," *1986/A Year in Nutritional Medicine Monograph*, Keats Publishing, Inc. New Canaan, Conn., p. 1, 1986.

4. Passwater, R.A. *The Antioxidants: The Nutrients That Guard Us Against Cancer, Heart Disease, Arthritis and Allergies-- And Even Slow the Aging Process*, Keats Publishing, Inc. New Canaan, Conn., p. 2, 1985.

5.  Bendich, A. "Antioxidant Micronutrients and Immune Response," *Micronutrients and Immune Functions*, Bendich, A. and Chandra, R.K. (eds.) *Annals N.Y. Academy of Sciences*, New York, 587:168, 1990.

6.  Diplock, A.T. "Antioxidant nutrients and disease prevention," *Am. J. Clin. Nutr.*, 53:189S-193S, 1991.

7.  Pryor, W.A. "Measurement of Oxidative Stress Status in Humans," *Cancer Epidemiology, Biomarker*, Vol. 7 and *Prevention*, Vol. 2, p. 289, 1993.

8.  Gutteridge, J.M. "Antioxidants, Nutritional Supplements, and Life-Threatening diseases," *British Journal of Biomedical Science*, Vol. 31, pp. 288-95. 1994.

9.  Ames, B.N. "Oxidants, Antioxidants, and the Degenerative Disease of Aging," *Proceedings of the National Academy of Science*, Vol. 90, pp. 7915-22, 1993.

10. Harman, D. "Free-Radical Theory of Aging: Increasing Functional Life Span," *Pharmacology of Aging Processes: Methods of Assessment and Potential Interventions in Annals of the New York Academy of Sciences*, Vol. 717, p. 1, 1994.

11. Voelker, R. "Radical Approaches: Is Widespread Testing and Treatment for Oxidative Injuries Coming Soon?" *JAMA*, Vol. 270, No. 17, p. 2024, 1993.

12. Richardson, S. "Free Radicals and Alzheimer's Disease," *Proceedings of the Alzheimer's*

*Association Annual Meeting, Research Update Session*, p. 13, 1992.

13. Harman, D. "Free-Radical Theory of Aging: Increasing the Functional Life Span," *Pharmacology of Aging Processes: Methods of Assessment and Potential Interventions in Annals of the New York Academy of Sciences*, Vol. 717, p. 5, 1994.

14. Carney, J. and A. "Role of Protein Oxidation in Aging and in Age-Associated Neurodegenerative Diseases," *Life Science*, Vol. 55, No. 25-26, pp. 1-7, 1994.

15. Smith, C.D., Carney, J.M., Tatsumo, T., et al. "Protein Oxidation in Aging Brain," *Annals of the New York Academy of Sciences: Aging and Cellular Defense Mechanism*, Vol. 663, pp. 110-19, 1993.

16. Diplock A.T. "Antioxidant Nutrients and Disease," *Nutrition and Health*, Vol. 9, pp. 37-42, 1993: N.D. Penn et al., "The Effect of Dietary Supplementation with Vitamins A, C, and E on Cell-Mediated Immune Function in Elderly Long-Stay Patients: A Randomized Controlled Trial" *Age and Aging*, Vol. 20, pp. 169-74, 1991.

17. Cooper, K.H. *Dr. Kennth H. Cooper's Antioxidant Revolution* (Nashville: Thomas Nelson), p. 119, 1994.

18. Chandra R.K. "Effect of Vitamin and Trace-Element Supplementation on Immune Responses and Infection in Elderly Subjects," *Lancet*, Vol. 340, pp. 1124-27, 1992.

19. Yanick, P., Jaffe, R. *Clinical Chemistry and Nutrition: A Physician's Desk Reference*, EPP, 1988.

20. Yanick, P. Dietary and Lifestyle Influences on Cochlear Disorders and Biochemical Status: A 12-month Study. *Journal of Applied Nutrition*, Vol. 40, no 2, 1988.

## CHAPTER 5:

1. Labrie C, Belanger A, Labrie F. Androgenic activity of dehydroepiandrosterone and androstenedione in the rat ventral prostate. Endocrinology. 123: 1412-1417, 1988.

2. Labrie F. Intracrinology. Mol Cell Endocrinol. 78:C113-C118, 1991.

3. Roy R, Belanger A. Lipoproteins: carriers of dehydroepiandrosterone fatty acid esters in human serum. J Steroid Biochem. 34:559-561, 1889.

4. Provencher PH, Roy R, Belanger A. Pregnenolone fatty acid esters incorporated into lipoproteins: substrates in adrenal steroidogenesis. Endocrinology. 130:2717-2724, 1992.

5. Roy R, Belanger A. 1989 Formation of lipoidal steroids in follicular fluid. J Steroid Biochem. 33:257-262, 1989.

6. Labrie F, Dupont A, Belanger A. Complete androgen blockade for the treatment of prostate cancer. In: De Vita Vt, Hellman S, Rosenberg SA, eds. Important advances in oncology. Philadelphia: Lippincott: 193-217, 1985.

7.  Brochu M, Belanger A, Dupont A, Cusan L, Labrie F. Effects of flutamide and aminoglutethimide on plasma 5a-reduced steroid glucuronide concentrations in castrated patients with cancer of the prostate. J Steroid Biochem. 28:619-622, 1987.

8.  Belanger A, Brochu M, Lacoste D, et al. Steroid glucuronides: human circulatory levels and formation by LNCaP cells. J Steroid Biochem Mol Biol. 40:593-598.

9.  Labrie F, Simard J, Luu-The V, Belanger A, Pelletier G. Structure, function and tissue-specific gene expression of 3b-hydroxysteroid dehydrogenase/5-ene-4-ene isomerase enzymes in classical and peripheral intracrine steroidogenic tissues. J Steroid Biochem Mol Biol. 43:805-826, 1992.

## CHAPTER 6:

1.  Unger RH. "Glucagon and the insulin: glucagon ratio in diabetes and other catabolic illnesses." Diabetes 20 834-838; 1971.

2.  Reaven GM. "Role of insulin resistance in human disease." Diabetes 37: 1595-1607; 1989.

3.  Rudman, D; Feller, A.G.; Nagraj, A.G.; et. al. "Effect of human growth hormone in men over 60 years old," *N. Eng. J. Med.* 323:1-9, 1990.

4.  Wolthers, T; Thorbjorn, G.; Lunde, J.O. "Effect of GH administration on functional hepatic

nitrogen clearance: studies in normal subjects and GH deficient patients," *J. Clin. Endocr. Metab.* 78:1220-24, 1994.

5. Rosen, T.; Johannsson, G.; Johnsson, J.; Bengtosson, B. "Consequences of growth hormone deficiency in adults and the benefits and risks of recombinant human growth hormone," *Horm. Res.* 43:93-99, 1995.

6. Papadeakis, M.A.; Grady D.: Black, D.; et. al. "Growth hormone replacement in healthy older men improves body composition but not functional ability," *Annals of Internal Medicine* 124:708-16, 1996.

7. Van Vollenhoven RF, Engleman EG, McGuire Jl. An open study of dehydroepiandrosterone in systemic lupus erthematosus. *Arthritis Rheum* 37:1305-1310; 1994.

8. Morales AJ, Nolan JJ, Nelson JC, Yen SS. Effects of replacement dose of dehydroepiandrosterone in men and women of advancing age. *J Clin Endocrinol Metab* 78:1360-1367; 1994.

9. Loviselli A, Pisanu P, Cossu E, et al. Low levels of dehydroepiandrosterone sulfate in adult males with insulin-dependent diabetes mellitus. *Minerva Endocrinol* 19:113-119; 1994.

10. Ebeling, Pertti; Koivisto, Veikko A. Physiological importance of dehydroepiandrosterone. *The Lancet*, v343 n8911 p1479 (3); 1994.

11. Yen SS, Morales AJ, Khorram O. Replacement of DHEA in aging men and women. Potential remedial effects. *Ann NY Acad Sci*, 774:128-142; 1995.

12. Turek, F.W. Melatonin Hype Hard to Swallow. *Nature* Vol. 379; 295-296: January 25, 1996.

13. Eblhara, S., Marks, T. Hudson, D.J. & Menaker M. *Science* 231, 491-493, 1986.

14. Elias, M. The mysteries of melatonin. *Harvard Health letter* 18(8):6(3); 1993.

15. Laakso, M. L.; Leinonen, L.; Hatonen, T.; Alila, A.; and Heiskala, H. Melatonin, Cortisol and body temperature.

**CHAPTER 7:**

1. Finch, Caleb E. *Longevity, Senescence and the Genome.* Chicago: University of Chicago Press, 1990.

2. Arking, Robert, *Biology of Aging: Observations and Principles.* Englewood Cliffs, N.J., Prentice Hall, 1991.

3. Branch, Laurence G., Jack M. Guralnik, Daniel J. Foley, Frank J. Kohout Terrie T. Wetle, Adrian Ostfeld, and Sidney Katz. "Active Life Expectancy for Ten Thousand Caucasian Men and Women in Three Communities." *Journal of Gerontology* 46 (1991): M145-50.

4. Kohn, Robert R. "Cause of Death in Very Old People." *Journal of American Medical Association* 247, no. 20 (1982):2793-97.

5. Manton, Kenneth G., Eric Stallard, and H. Dennis Tolley. "Limits to Human Life Expectancy: Evidence, Prospects, and Implications." *Population and Development Review* 17 (December 1991):603-36.

6.  "An Aging World II," U.S. Bureau of the Census, International Population Reports, P25, 92-3, U.S. Government Printing Office, Washington D.C., 1992.

7.  Scheer, J.F. Vitamin E: Our Prime Protectant. *"Better nutrition for Today's Living"*, Vol. 56, 1994.

8.  Cavenee, W. and While, R. The Genetic Basis of Cancer, *Scientfic American*, March, 1995.

9.  Kartner, N. and Ling, V. Multidrug Resistance in Cancer, *Scientific American*, 1993.

10. Lahkovsky, G. *Radiations and Waves: Sources of our Life*, E.L. Cabella, NY, 1941.

11. McClare, C.W.F., "Resonance in Bioenergetics", Annals of NY Acad. Sciences. 227: 74-91, 1974.

12. Rapp, P.R., "An Atlas of Cellular Oscillators", *Journ. Of Exp. Biology*, 81: 281-306, 1979.

13. Popp, F.A. *Electromagnetic Bio-Information, Urban and Schwartzenburg*, 1989.

14. Omura, Y. Connections between each Meridian, Hormones unique to each Meridian, etc. Acupuncture & Electro-Therapeutics Res., Int. J. Vol. 14, Pergamon Press. 1989.

15. Martiny, M. "Opotherapie et homeopathie" *Homeopath*. Mod., 5,8 :123-529, 1936.

16. Pischinger, A. *Matrix and Matrix Regulation*, Haug Publishers. 1991.

17. Royal, F. Fuller, "Understanding Homeopathy, Acupuncture and Electrodiagnosis: Clinical

Applications of Quantum Mechanics," *American Journal of Acupuncture* 18(1):37-53, 1990.

18. Schimmel, H.W. *Basic Pathogenic Patterns and Causal Chains*, Pascoe, 1991.

19. Brumer, P. and Shapiro, M. Laser Control of Chemical Reactions, *Scientific American*, March, 1995.

20. Englert et al. *Scientific American*, 1994.

21. Becker, R. *Cross Currents*. Jeremy Tarcher, Inc. 1990.

22. Wilson, B.W., Wright, C., and Anderson, L.E. "Evidence for an Effect of ELF Electromagnetic Fields on Human Pineal Gland Function." *Journal of Pineal Research* 9: 259-69; 1990.

23. Semm, P., Schneider, T., and Vollrath, L. "Effects of an Earth-Strength Magnetic Field on Electrical Activity of Pineal Cells." *Nature* 288: 607-8; 1980.

24. Wilson, B.W., Stevens, R.G., and Anderson, L.E. "Neuroendocrine Mediated Effects of Electromagnetic-Field Exposure: Possible Role of the Pineal Gland." *Life Sciences* 45: 1319-32; 1989.

25. Dubbels, R., Klenke, E., Manz, B., Terwey, J., and Schloot, W. "Melatonin Determination with a Newly Developed ELISA System. Interindividual Differences in the Response of the Human Pineal Gland to Magnetic Fields." *Advances in Pineal Research*, vol. 7, ed. G.J. Maestroni, A. Conti, and R.J. Reiter (London: John Libbey and Co.,), pp. 27-33; 1994.

26. "Correlation Between Heart Attacks and Magnetic Activity." *Nature* 277:646-48; 1994.

## CHAPTER 8:

1.  Yanick, P. "Physiological-Chemical Assessment of Undernutrition" *Townsend Letter for Doctors*, July, 1988.

2.  Yanick, P. "Biomolecular Nutrition and the GI Tract" *Townsend Letter for Doctors*, Dec., 1993.

3.  Yanick, P. Dietary and Lifestyle Influences on Cochlear Disorders and Biochemical Status: A 12-month study. *Journal of Applied Nutrition*, Vol. 40, no. 2, 1988.

4.  Yanick, P., Jaffee, R. *Clinical Chemistry and Nutrition: A Physician's Desk Reference*, EPP, 1988.

5.  Yanick, P. "Functional Medicine Update" *Townsend Letter for Doctors*, Feb., 1994.

6.  Yanick, P. *Bioregulation, Regeneration and Lifespan Extension.* Yanick, Inc. 1994.

7.  Adibi, S., Phillips E: Evidence for greater absorption of amino acids from peptide than from free form in human intestine. *Clin Res*, 16:446, 1968.

8.  Craft, I.L., Geddes, D., Hyde, C.W., et al: Absorption and malabsorption of glycine and glycine peptides in man. *Gut* 9:425-437, 1968.

9.  Adibi, S.A., Fogel, M.R., Agrawal R.M. Comparison of free amino acid and dipeptide

absorption in the jejunum of sprue patients. *Gastroenterology* 67: 586-591, 1974.

10. Reicht, G., Petritsch, W., Eherer, A., et al: Jejunal protein absorption of whey protein and its hydrolysate. *JPEN*, 16:25S, 1992.

11. Neredith J.W., Ditesheim, J.A., Zaloga G.P. Visceral protein levels in trauma patients are greater with peptide diet than intact protein diet. *J Trauma*, 30:825-829, 1990.

12. Gardner, M.G. Intestinal assimilation of intact peptides and proteins from the diet—A neglected field. *Biol Rev* 59:289-331, 1984.

13. Boullin, D.J., Crampton, R.F., Heading, C.E. et al: Intestinal absorption of dipeptides containing glycine, phenylalanine, proline, B-alanine, or histidine in the rat. *Clinical Science Molecular Medicine* 45:849-858, 1973.

14. Gardner, M.G. Absorption of intact peptides— Studies on transport of protein digest and dipeptides across rat small intestine in vitro. *Q J Exp Physiol* 67:629-637, 1982.

15. Webb, K.E. Amino acid and peptide absorption from the gastrointestinal tract. *Federation Proceeding* 45:2268-2271, 1986.

16. Amoss, M., Rivier. J., Guillemin, R. Release of gonadotropins by oral administration of synthetic LRF or a tripeptide fragment of LRF. *J Clin Endocrinol Metab* 35:175-177, 1972.

17. Bowers, C.Y., Schally, A.V., Enzmann, F., et al: Porcine thyrotrophin releasing hormone is

(pyro)Glu-His-Pro(NH2). *Endocrinology* 86:1143-1153, 1970.

18. Gardner, M.L.G. Entry of peptides of dietary origin into the circulation. *Nutr Health* 2:163-171, 1983.

19. Adibi, S.A. Intestinal absorption of dipeptides in man: Relative importance of hydrolysis and intact absorption. *J Clin Invest* 50:2266-2275, 1971.

20. Newey, H., Smyth, D.H. The intestinal absorption of some dipeptides. *J Physiol* 145:48-56, 1959.

21. Perry, T.L., Hansen, S., Tischler, B., et al: A new metabolic disorder associated with neurological disease and mental defect. *N Engl J Med* 277:1219-1227, 1967.

22. Zaloga, G.P., Chernow, B., Zajtchuk, R., et al: Diagnostic dosages of protirelin (TRH) elevate blood pressure by noncatecholamine mechanisms. Arch Intern Med 144:1149-1152.

23. Bounous, G., Kongshavn P.A.L. Influence of dietary proteins on the immune system of mice. *J Nutr* 112:1747-1755, 1982.

24. Rouse, I.L., Beilin, L.J. Vegetarian diet and blood pressure. *J Hypertension* 2:2331-240, 1984.

25. Kontessis, P., Jones, S., Dodds, R., et al: Renal, metabolic and hormonal responses to ingestion of animal and vegetable proteins. *Kidney Int* 38:136-144, 1990.

26. Silk, D.B.A., Fairclough, P.D., Clark, M.L., et al: Use of a peptide rather than free amino nitrogen source in chemically defined "elemental" diets. *JPEN* 4:548-553, 1980.

27. Keohane P.P., Grimble, G.K., Brown, B., et al: Influence of protein composition and hydrolysis method on intestinal absorption of protein in man. *Gut* 26:907-913, 1985.

28. Sears B. "Essential fatty acids and dietary endocronology." *J. Adv. Med.* 6: 211-224; 1993.

29. Willis Al. "Handbook of Eiosanoids, Prostglandins and Related Lipids," CRC Press. Boca Raton, FL; 1987.

30. Bergstrom S, Rhyhage R, Samuelsson B, and Sorval J. "The Structure of prostaglandins E1, E1a and F1B," *J. Biol. Chem.* 238: 3555-3565; 1963.

31. Sinclair A and Gibson R. "Essential Fatty Acids and Eiosanoids," *Amer. Oil Chem, Soc.* Champaign, IL; 1992.

32. Brenner RR. "Nutrition and hormonal factors influencing desaturation of essential fatty acids." *Prog. Lipid Res.* 20: 41-48; 1982.

33. Diplock, A.T. "Antioxidant nutrients and disease prevention," *Am. J. Nutr.*, 53:p. 190S, 1991.

34. Ali, M. Nutritional Medicine: Principles and Practice, Institute of Preventive Medicine, Denville, N.J., 1991.

35. Jacques, P.F., Taylor, A. "Micronutrients and Age-Related Cataracts," in *Micronutrients in Health and in Disease Prevention*, Bendich, A., Butterworth, C.E., (eds.), Marcel Dekker, New York, pp. 359-379, 1991.

36. Bobyre, V.N., Vese'lski, I. Sh., Bobyreva, L.E. "Antioxidants in the Prevention and Treatment of

Cerebral Arteriosclerosis," *Zh. Nevropatol. Piskhiatr.*, 89(9): p. 60-3, 1989.

37. Lonsdale, D. "Free Oxygen Radicals and Disease," in *1986/A Year in Nutritional Medicine Monograph*, Keats Publishing, Inc., New Canaan, Conn., p. 14, 1986.

38. Nardi, E.A., et al., "High-dose reduced glutathione in the therapy of alcoholic hepatopathy," *Clin. Ter.*, 136(1):47-51, January 15, 1991.

39. Bresci, G. et al., "The Use of Reduced Glutathione in Alcoholic Hepatopathy," *Minera. Med.*, 82(11): 753-55, November 1991.

40. Levy, D.I. "Glutahione prevent N-methyl-D-asparate receptor-mediated neurotoxicity," *Neuroreport*, 2(6): 345-47, June, 1991.

**CHAPTER 9:**

1. Campbell, T. C. *"A Plant-Enriched Diet and Long-term Health, Particularly in Reference to China."* Paper presented at the Second International Symposium on Horticulture and Human Health, Alexandria, VA. (November 4, 1989).

2. Campbell, T. C. et al., "China: From Diseases of Poverty to Diseases of Affluence. Policy Implications of the Epidemiological Transition." Paper part of NIH Grant 5R01CA33638 (Bethesda, Md.: *National Institutes of Health*, 1990).

3.  Ornish, D. et al., "Can Lifestyle Changes Reverse Coronary Heart Disease? (The Life-Style Heart Trial)," *The Lancet* 336 129-133; 1990.

4.  Ellis, F. R. et al., "Incidence of Osteoporosis in Vegetarians and Ommivores," *American Journal of Clinical Nutrition* 6 555-558;1972.

5.  Stokkan, K.A.; Reiter, R.J.; Nonaka, K,O.; et al. Food restriction retards aging of the pineal gland. *Brain Res.* 545:66-72, 1991.

6.  Young V. R. and Pellett, P. L., "Protein Intake and Requirements with Reference to Diet and Health," *American Journal of Clinical Nutrition* 45 1323-1343; 1987.

7.  Weindruch, R. and Walford, R. L. *The Retardation of Aging and Disease by Dietary Restriction.* Charles C Thomas, Springfield, IL, 1988.

8.  Yanick, P. Dietary and Lifestyle Influences on Cochlear Disorders and Biochemical Status: A 12-month study. *Journal of Applied Nutrition*, Vol. 40, no. 2, 1988.

9.  Unger RH. "Glucagon and the insulin: glucagon ratio in diabetes and other catabolic illnesses." *Diabetes* 20 834-838; 1971.

10. Reaven GM. "Role of insulin resistance in human disease." *Diabetes* 37: 1595-1607; 1989

11. Galbo H, Holst J, and Christensen NJ. "The effect of different diets of insulin on the hormonal response to prolonged exercise." *Acta Physiol Scand.* 107: 19-32; 1979

12. Brenner RR. "Nutrition and hormonal factors influencing desaturation of essential fatty acids." *Prog. Lipid Res.* 20: 41-48; 1982

13. Samuelsson B. "On incorporation of oxygen in the conversion of 8, 11, 14 eicoatrienoic acid into prostaglandin E." *J. Am. Chem. Soc.* 89: 3011-3013; 1965.

14. Sears B. "Essential fatty acids and dietary endocrinology." *J. Adv. Med.* 6: 211-224; 1993.

15. Sinclair A and Gibson R. "Essential Fatty Acids and Eicosanoids," *Amer. Oil Chem, Soc.* Champaign, IL; 1992.

## CHAPTER 10:

1. Monroe, R.A. *Ultimate Journey*, New York: Doubleday, 1994.

2. Russell, R. *Using The Whole Brain*, Hampton Roads Publishing Company, Inc., 1993.

## CHAPTER 11:

1. Harley, N.W., Kim, K.R., Prowse, S.L., Weinrich, K.S., Hirsch, M.D., West, S., Bacchetti, H.W., Hirte, C.W., Greider, W.E., Wright, J.W. *Telomerase, Cell Immortality and Cancer*. Shay in Cold spring Harbor Symposia in Quantitative Biology, Vol. LVIX, Pages 307-315, 1994.

2. Greider, C.W. and Blackburn, E.H. *Telomeres, Telomerase and Cancer*. Scientific American. 1996.

3. Boon, T. *Teaching the Immune System To Fight Cancer*. Scientific American, 1993.

4. Chang, E. and Harley, C.B. "Telomere Length as a Measure of Replicative Histories in Human Vascular Tissues," *Proceedings of the National Academy of Science*, Vol. 92, 1995.

5. DiGiovanna, A.G. *Human Aging: Biological Perspectives*. New York: McGraw-Hill, 1994.

6. Fackelmann, K. "Protein Protects, Restores Neurons." *Science News*, Vol. 147, p. 52, 1995.

7. Haber, D.A. "Telomeres, Cancer and Immortality." *New England Journal of Medicine*, Vol. 332, pp. 95-96, 1995.

8. Kim, N.W., et al. "Specific Association of Human Telomerase Activity with Immortal Cells and Cancer." *Science*, Vol. 266, pp. 2001-14, 1994.

9. Marx, J. "How a Cell Cycles Toward Cancer." *Science*, Vol. 263, pp. 319-321, 1994.

10. Service, R.F. "Dendrimers: Dream Molecules Approach Real Applications." *Science*, Vol. 267, pp. 458-59, 1995.

11. Schneider, E.L. *Genetics of Aging*. New York: Plenum, 1978.

# INDEX

## A

# D

# E